Easy French
FOR BEGINNERS

Tired of the struggle to learn a new language? Still traumatized by school teachers?

Don't let the past hold you back! Make learning French fun & easy with our bilingual books!

"EASY FRENCH FOR BEGINNERS" includes vocab, grammar, fun games, & quizzes.

SAY GOODBYE TO STRUGGLES AND HELLO TO FLUENCY! GET YOUR COPY NOW

nook   kobo   INGRAM   BARNES & NOBLE Booksellers   iBooks   amazon.com

WWW.BILINGUALBOOKSTORE.COM

Pump it up Magazine

TABLE OF CONTENTS

⚡ **Letter from The Editor** — 5
Anissa Sutton

⚡ **CUSTOM CAR SECRETS**
Paint, Gear & Garage Tips Every Man Should Know

⚡ **WELLNESS** — 21
Best Superfoods For energy & immunity

⚡ **BEST THRILLERS** — 30
To Keep You on the Edge of Your Seat

⚡ **QUIZ**
Do You Have Mental Strength?

⚡ **COVER STORY SOLO ELEMENT**
#1 Award-Winning Custom Airbrush Car Artist in Los Angeles

⚡ **BUILD YOUR GARAGE GYM** — 11
Strength Hacks for Busy Men
Fatherhood & Fitness

⚡ **LOWRIDER LIFE & LOCAL LOVE**
Where Cars, Music & Food Bring Us Together

⚡ **HUMANITARIAN AWARENESS**
Drive & Donate: 6 Easy Ways to Show Love & Support
Support artists & local communities — donate, attend, or share!

Reach for the Stars - While Standing on Earth!

Pump it up MAGAZINE ®

PUMP IT UP MAGAZINE
LINKS

WEBSITE
www.pumpitupmagazine.com

FACEBOOK
www.facebook.com/pumpitupmagazine

TWITTER
www.twitter.com/pumpitupmag

SOUNDCLOUD
www.soundcloud.com/pumpitupmagazine

INSTAGRAM
pumpitupmagazine

PINTEREST
www.pinterest.com/pumpitupmagazine

PUMP IT UP MAGAZINE
30721 Russell Ranch Road
Suite 140
Westlake Village,
California 91362
United States
www.pumpitupmagazine.com
info@pumpitupmagazine.com
Tel : (001) (877)841 – 7414 (toll free number)

EDITORIAL

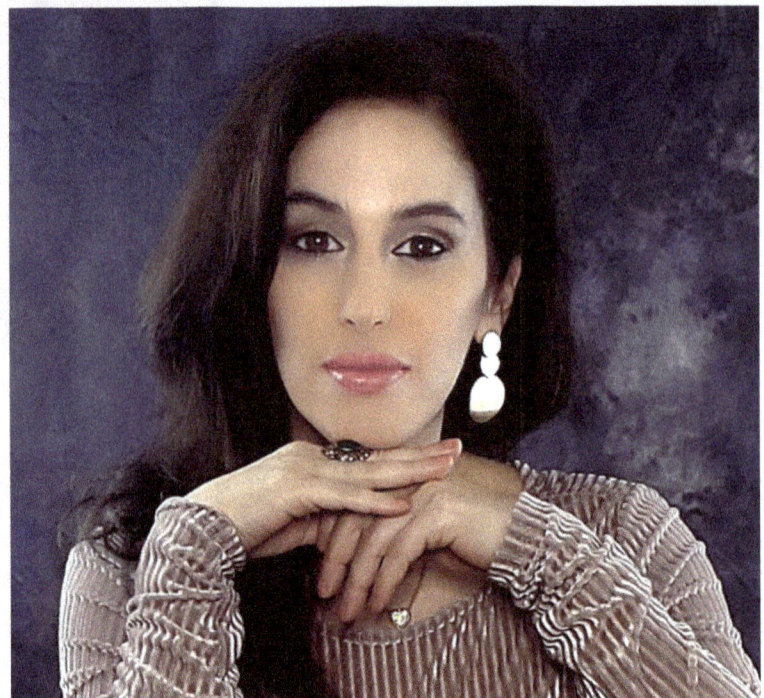

Greetings Readers,

Welcome to a new issue—an issue full of real people, bold moves, big dreams, and even bigger hearts.

When we first started Pump It Up Magazine, I wanted to create something more than just pages filled with pretty pictures or passing trends. I wanted a place where voices could be heard, where underdogs could shine, and where strength looked like resilience, not perfection.

This issue? It's proof that the streets talk—and we listen.

From the custom brilliance of Solo Element, turning steel and paint into stories, to f dads building garage gyms, and lowrider culture that unites generations—this edition is all about power in motion. Whether it's the bounce of hydraulics, the rhythm of soul and funk, or the steady pulse of wellness and purpose… it all comes down to this: movement.

And while the world keeps racing, we're here to remind you—it's okay to slow down reflect, and reclaim your joy. Maybe it's in a playlist, maybe in a workout, maybe in a moment of stillness. Whatever it is, hold onto it.

Because your life? It's art.
Your journey? Worth every page.
Your voice? We're listening.

We keep sharing, we keep growing, and we keep Pumpin' It Up—together.
So flip through with love.
Highlight your favorites.
Share them with someone who needs a little spark.

We're just getting started—and we're so glad you're here with us.

With love and good vibes,
Be safe and be blessed!!

Anissa Boudjaoui Sutton

CONTRIBUTORS

PUBLISHER EDITOR
Editions L.A.
AnissaSutton.com

MUSIC
Michael B. Sutton

MARKETING
Grace Rose
Shaun Brown

PARTNERS

Editions L.A.
www.editions-la.com

The Sound Of L.A.
www.thesoundofla.com

Info Music
www.infomusic.fr

YMC
yourmusicconsultant.com

Magazine Cover
Mark Maryanovich

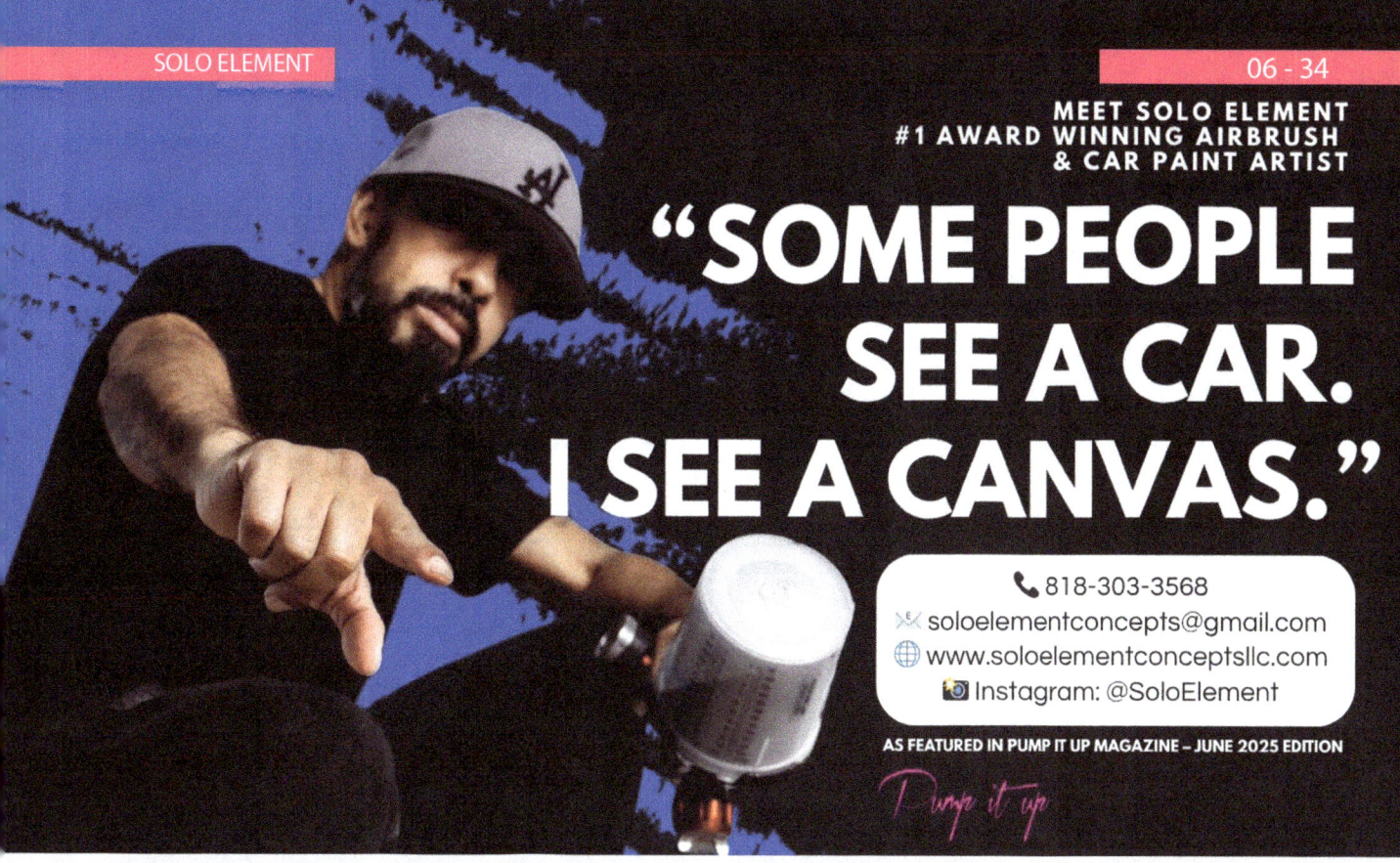

**MEET SOLO ELEMENT
#1 AWARD WINNING AIRBRUSH
& CAR PAINT ARTIST**

"SOME PEOPLE SEE A CAR. I SEE A CANVAS."

📞 818-303-3568
✉ soloelementconcepts@gmail.com
🌐 www.soloelementconceptsllc.com
📷 Instagram: @SoloElement

AS FEATURED IN PUMP IT UP MAGAZINE – JUNE 2025 EDITION

Pump it up

Some people see a car. Reinaldo Fuentes, aka Solo Element, sees a canvas.
And what he creates is nothing short of rolling art in motion.

As the founder of Solo Element Concepts LLC, Fuentes has redefined what custom car paint means in Los Angeles — transforming raw steel into bold, personal expressions of identity and pride.

"This isn't just a paint job," Fuentes says. "It's a reflection of who you are. I want people to feel proud, confident, and stylish every time they drive away."

Raised in Caguas, Puerto Rico, Solo Element's journey began at just 10 years old, when his mother gifted him his first airbrush. By 15, he was painting full cars, laying the foundation for the award-winning career that would eventually bring him to Los Angeles.

"'Solo' represents individuality," he explains. "'Element' is where I come alive creatively."

From vibrant lowriders and high-gloss muscle cars to motorcycles, surfboards, and guitars, Solo Element brings his precise airbrush techniques to nearly any surface. Each project begins with a conversation, turning every client's story into a one-of-a-kind design.

One standout? A full mural inspired by Don Quixote, meticulously painted after reading the book and studying the character's journey. Every flame, every detail carries

His work has earned top honors across the custom car industry:

Best of Show – Slamfest 2012 & Classic Orlando 2012

Best Paint & Interior – Dub Show Miami 2013

Features in Baggers Magazine, Mustang Magazine, and appearances at the legendary SEMA Show Las Vegas.

Beyond cars, Solo Element's artistry extends to surfboards and musical instruments, blending his passion for detail with storytelling across every surface.

"At the end of the day, it's all a canvas — whether it's metal, wood, or fiberglass. I want people to feel pride and identity in everything they ride, drive, or play."

Ready to PUMP UP Your Ride?
Solo Element is ready to bring your vision to life.

📞 818-303-3568
✉ soloelementconcepts@gmail.com
🌐 www.soloelementconceptsllc.com
📷 Instagram: @SoloElement

SOLO ELEMENT

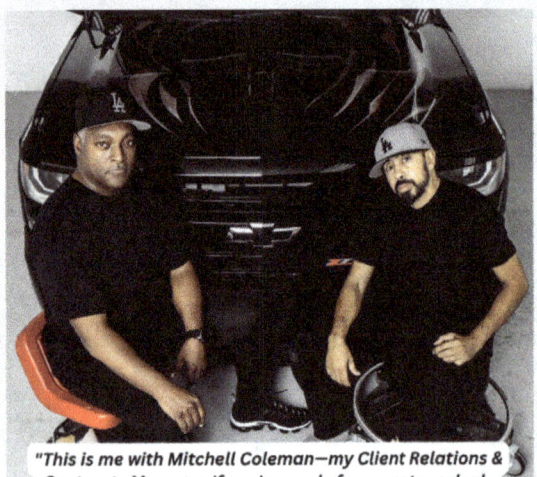

"This is me with Mitchell Coleman—my Client Relations & Contracts Manager. If you're ready for a quote, a deal, or to get your custom ride started, hit us up. Call now: 818-303-3568. Let's make your vision real."

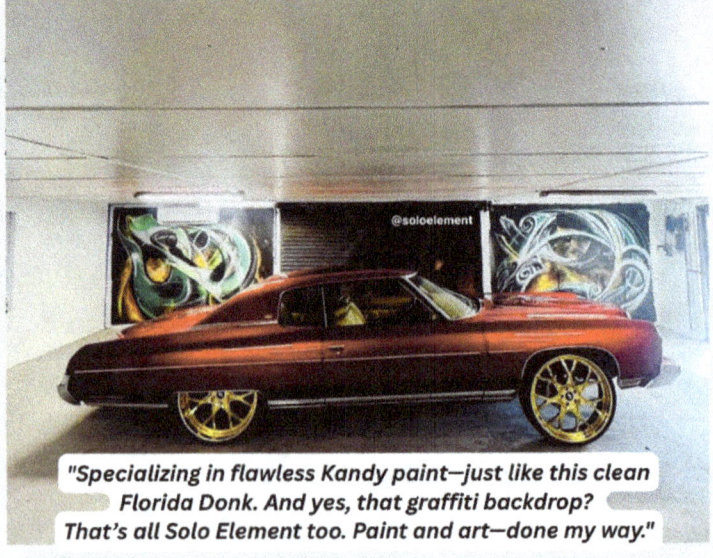

"Specializing in flawless Kandy paint—just like this clean Florida Donk. And yes, that graffiti backdrop? That's all Solo Element too. Paint and art—done my way."

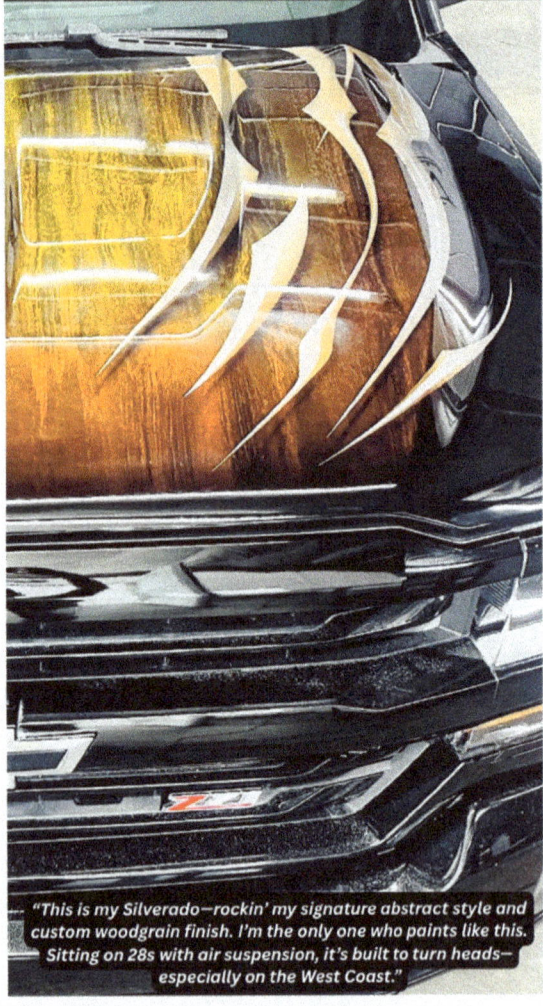

"This is my Silverado—rockin' my signature abstract style and custom woodgrain finish. I'm the only one who paints like this. Sitting on 28s with air suspension, it's built to turn heads—especially on the West Coast."

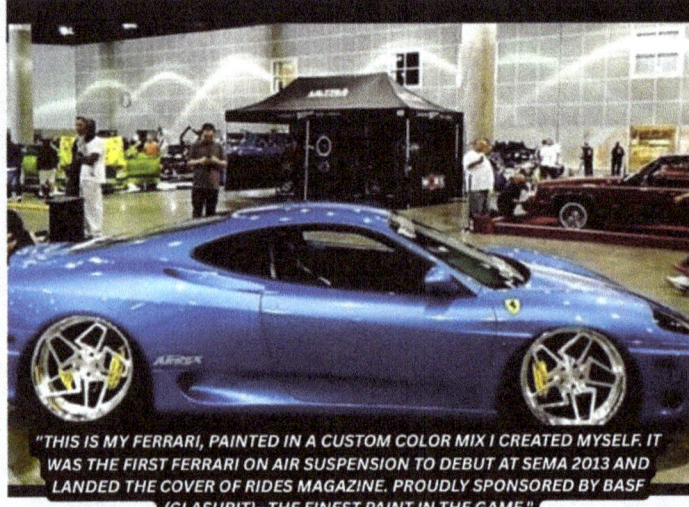

"THIS IS MY FERRARI, PAINTED IN A CUSTOM COLOR MIX I CREATED MYSELF. IT WAS THE FIRST FERRARI ON AIR SUSPENSION TO DEBUT AT SEMA 2013 AND LANDED THE COVER OF RIDES MAGAZINE. PROUDLY SPONSORED BY BASF (GLASURIT)—THE FINEST PAINT IN THE GAME."

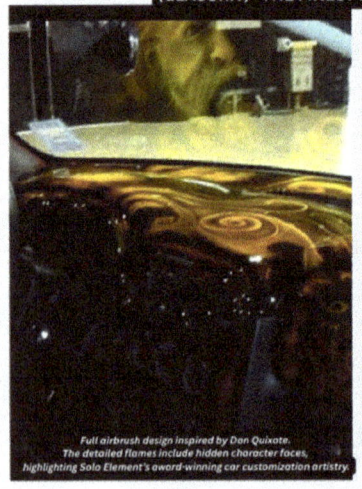

Full airbrush design inspired by Don Quixote. The detailed flames include hidden character faces, highlighting Solo Element's award-winning car customization artistry.

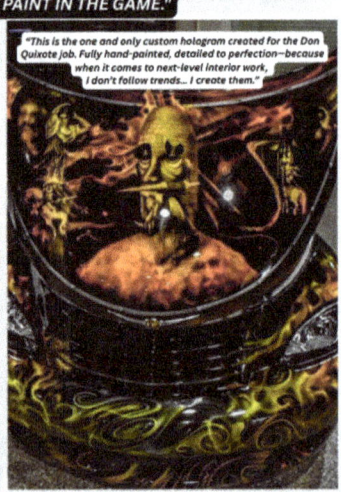

"This is the one and only custom hologram created for the Don Quixote job. Fully hand-painted, detailed to perfection—because when it comes to next-level interior work, I don't follow trends... I create them."

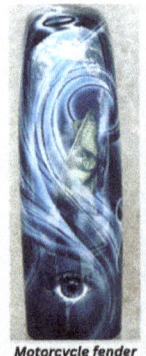

Motorcycle fender with realistic dollar bill

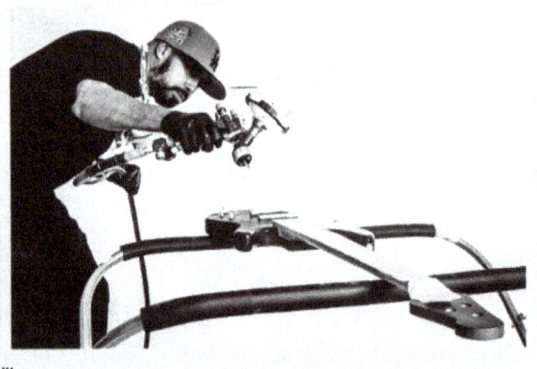

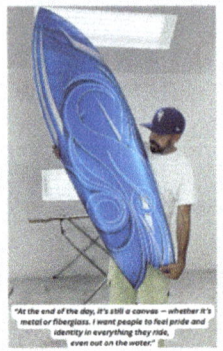

"At the end of the day, it's still a canvas — whether it's metal or fiberglass. I want people to feel pride and identity in everything they ride, even out on the water."

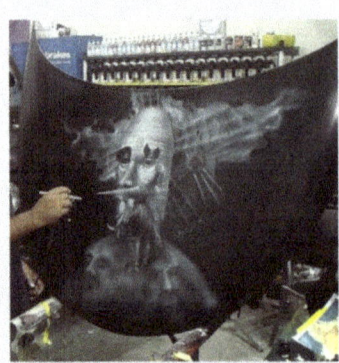

SOLO ELEMENT

PIUM: Let's start with your story. Where are you from, and how did this journey begin for you?

SOLO ELEMENT: I'm from Caguas, Puerto Rico. My journey started when I was 10 years old. My mother—an artist herself—recognized that I had the same spark early on. One Christmas, she gave me an airbrush, and that was the beginning. By the time I was 15, my father got me a summer job at an autobody shop to keep me out of trouble. That's where I painted my first car. It came naturally—I was able to combine my airbrush and paintbrush skills, and I've never looked back.

PIUM: What inspired you to turn your passion into a full-time business?

SOLO ELEMENT: I was deeply inspired by the custom paintwork I saw in Lowrider Magazine. Seeing artists bring their vision to life on cars made me realize: I could do that too—and make it my way of life.

PIUM: What does "Solo Element Concepts" represent, and how did the name come to life?

SOLO ELEMENT: "Solo Element" is a reflection of who I am and how I live. "Solo" represents being an individual, and "Element" is about being in your zone—your space of happiness and creativity. Together, it means being that one person who thrives in his element. That's how I approach every project.

PIUM: What kinds of vehicles do you customize—and how do you approach each one differently?

SOLO ELEMENT: I'm completely self-taught, so I don't follow a textbook method. Many clients don't know the steps it takes to get to the final result—they just know how they want it to feel. My role is to step into their imagination, extract their vision, and transform it into something they didn't even realize was possible.

PIUM: Tell us about a project that really impacted you.

SOLO ELEMENT: There was a customer who brought me a novel and asked me to read it. It was Don Quixote. He had me watch a play and listen to music inspired by the story. He and his wife would come watch me paint scenes from the book, live. My art told the story. That project stayed with me because it challenged me on every level—and connected me deeply to the character's journey. It was storytelling through paint.

PIUM: Where do you find inspiration for your designs and details?

SOLO ELEMENT: Inspiration comes from the client's story. Their memories, their dreams, their style—that's what I build around.

PIUM: What do you hope people feel when they drive away in one of your custom builds?

SOLO ELEMENT: I want them to feel proud, confident, and stylish. Like they're in something one-of-a-kind that reflects who they are. It's not just a paint job—it's a piece of them.

PIUM: What advice would you give someone dreaming of a career like yours?

SOLO ELEMENT: Be confident. Stay focused. Don't chase the money—perfect your craft. When you truly do what you love, the money will follow.

PIUM: And finally, how can people reach you to start their transformation?

SOLO ELEMENT: You can reach me through my website www.soloelementconceptsllc.com or call me directly 818-303-3568. I'm always ready to help bring your vision to life.

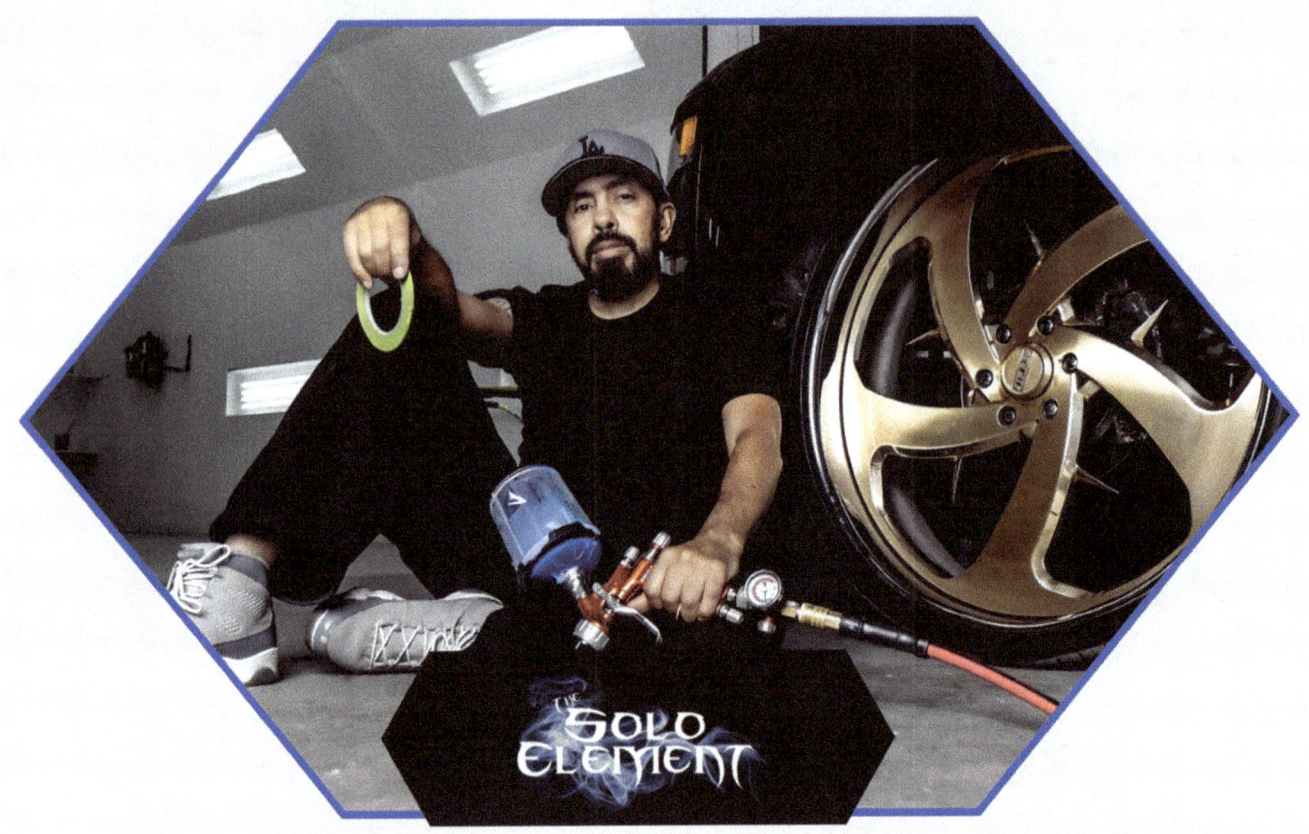

DECORATING THE STREET

Full Custom Paint Jobs

Airbrush Art & Graphics

Flake & Candy Finishes

Pinstriping & Detailing

Classic Repaints

One-of-One Designs

**LET'S BUILD YOUR DREAM RIDE!
CONTACT SOLO TODAY.**

SCAN TO WATCH!

 818-303-3568   WWW.SOLOELEMENTCONCEPTSLLC.COM

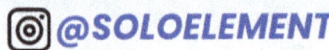 @SOLOELEMENT

TIPS FOR STAYING ACTIVE AND FITS

Staying active and maintaining fitness are essential components of a healthy lifestyle. Whether you're new to exercising or a seasoned athlete, incorporating regular physical activity into your daily routine can boost your physical health, mental well-being, and overall quality of life. Here are some practical tips to help you stay active and fit:

1. Set Realistic Goals
Setting achievable goals is crucial for staying motivated. Start with small, attainable objectives and gradually increase your intensity and duration. For example, if you're new to fitness, aim for a 15-minute walk three times a week and gradually increase the time and frequency.

2. Find an Activity You Enjoy
The key to staying active is finding an exercise you enjoy. Whether it's dancing, swimming, hiking, or cycling, choosing an activity that you look forward to will make it easier to stick with it. Variety can also keep your routine exciting and engaging.

3. Incorporate Strength Training
Strength training is vital for building muscle, boosting metabolism, and preventing injury. Include exercises like push-ups, squats, and weightlifting in your routine at least twice a week. Remember to start with lighter weights and gradually increase as you build strength.

4. Stay Consistent
Consistency is critical to achieving and maintaining fitness. Try to incorporate physical activity into your daily routine, whether taking the stairs instead of the elevator, walking during lunch breaks, or scheduling regular workout sessions.

5. Monitor Your Progress
Tracking your progress can provide motivation and help you stay on track. Keep a journal or use a fitness app to record your workouts, track improvements, and celebrate milestones.

6. Prioritize Nutrition
A balanced diet is essential for supporting your fitness goals. Eat plenty of fruits, vegetables, lean proteins, and whole grains. Stay hydrated by drinking plenty of water, and consider consulting with a nutritionist for personalized advice.

7. Listen to Your Body
It's crucial to listen to your body and avoid overexertion. Rest days are as important as workout days, allowing your muscles to recover and preventing burnout. If you experience pain or discomfort, consult with a healthcare professional.

8. Stay Accountable
Having a workout buddy or joining a fitness group can provide accountability and support. Sharing your goals and progress with others can motivate you to stay committed to your fitness journey.

9. Mix Up Your Routine
Prevent boredom and plateaus by varying your workouts. Try new activities, such as yoga, pilates, or martial arts. This not only keeps things interesting but also challenges different muscle groups.

10. Make Fitness Fun
Incorporate fun into your fitness routine by setting challenges, rewarding yourself for reaching milestones, or trying new sports and activities. The more enjoyable your workouts, the more likely you will stick with them.

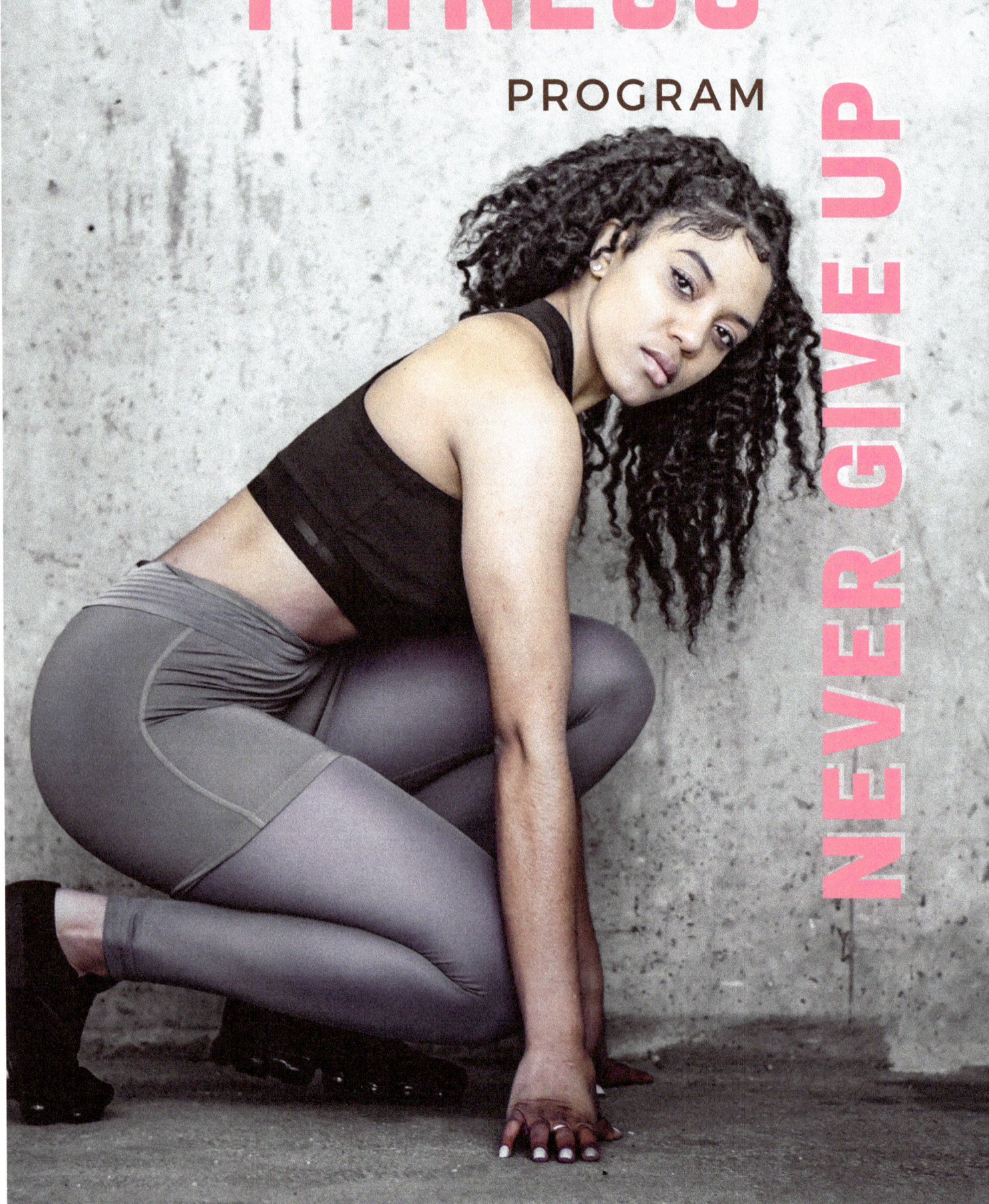

BUILD YOUR GARAGE GYM: STRENGTH HACKS FOR BUSY MEN
CONQUER YOUR SCHEDULE. BUILD YOUR BODY. NO EXCUSES.

For the modern man juggling work, family, and everything in between, finding time to hit the gym can feel like an impossible feat. But what if your fitness sanctuary was just a few steps away—in your own garage? With a smart setup and the right hacks, your garage gym can become a powerhouse of strength and discipline.

1. START SMALL, GO HEAVY

You don't need a full commercial setup to build real muscle. Focus on the essentials:

Barbell + Plates
Adjustable Dumbbells
Flat Bench
Pull-Up Bar

With just these basics, you can perform compound lifts like deadlifts, squats, presses, and rows—movements that give you the most bang for your buck.

2. TIME-SAVING PROGRAMMING

Forget the 90-minute gym marathons. Opt for 30–40 minute sessions using:
Supersets (e.g., bench + rows)
EMOMs (Every Minute on the Minute) for cardio and conditioning
5x5 or Push-Pull-Legs Split for structure

Efficiency is the name of the game. Strength doesn't require long hours—just consistency and intensity.

3. USE WHAT YOU'VE GOT

Got a tire, sledgehammer, or sandbag? Perfect. These non-traditional tools build functional strength and explosiveness. Plus, they're fun and primal—ideal for high-intensity sessions.

4. MAKE IT MOTIVATING

Paint the walls, hang a whiteboard with your goals, blast your playlist. Your garage gym should pump you up the second you walk in. Add a fan or heater so temperature isn't an excuse.

5. SET BOUNDARIES & SCHEDULE IT

This is your time. Treat your garage workouts like a meeting with your future self. Block off 3–5 slots per week in your calendar—even if it's 6am or 9pm. You'll thank yourself later.

FINAL WORD:
You don't need a fancy gym or expensive equipment—just grit, focus, and a corner of your garage. Build your temple. Build your strength. No more waiting for a better time.

WANT MORE TIPS ON BUILDING THE ULTIMATE GARAGE GYM?
Want more tips on building the ultimate garage gym?
Visit www.pumpitupmagazine.com/top-tips
Get featured: info@pumpitupmagazine.com

BRADY "BAM BAM" HIESTAND

PROFESSIONAL TUF, UFC, MMA FIGHTER.

- Consistency: Train regularly to build and maintain skills.
- Balanced Training: Mix disciplines like BJJ, Muay Thai, and boxing.
- Strength & Conditioning: Enhance physical endurance and strength.
- Healthy Diet: Eat well to fuel training and recovery.
- Mental Toughness: Use visualization and meditation for focus.
- Practice: Regular sparring and drilling to refine techniques.
- Recovery: Prioritize rest to stay in peak condition.
- Support Network: Rely on family, friends, and coaches.
- Pre-Event Rituals: Establish calming routines.
- Motivation: Find what energizes you, like music.
- Opponent Analysis: Study others to develop strategies.
- Adaptability: Stay open to learning and evolving.

Get inspired and elevate your game with Brady Hiestand's top tips for success, designed to pump you up and help you achieve greatness both in and out of the ring.

www.pumpitupmagazine.com
@PUMPITUPMAGAZINE

TOP SONGS TO BOOST YOUR WORKOUT MOTIVATION

Music is an excellent motivator during workouts, providing the energy and rhythm needed to power through even the toughest routines. Here are some top songs to include in your workout playlist:

1. "Eye of the Tiger" by Survivor
This classic anthem is perfect for getting pumped up and ready to tackle any workout challenge.

2. "Can't Stop the Feeling!" by Justin Timberlake
An upbeat and positive track that will keep you moving and grooving throughout your workout.

3. "Stronger" by Kanye West
With its powerful message and energetic beat, this song is ideal for pushing through tough workouts.

4. "Uptown Funk" by Mark Ronson ft. Bruno Mars
This funky and catchy tune is great for cardio or dance-based exercises, keeping your energy high.

5. "Lose Yourself" by Eminem
Eminem's intense lyrics and strong beat make this track perfect for staying focused and motivated.

6. "Don't Stop the Music" by Rihanna
A great track for keeping your rhythm and energy levels up, perfect for any cardio workout.

7. "Square Biz" by Funk Therapy feat. Victoria Renée
A vibrant cover of Teena Marie's classic hit, "Square Biz" brings a fresh, energetic vibe perfect for workouts. Victoria Renée's powerful vocals and the funky beats make this song a must-have for any playlist, keeping you energized and motivated.

8. "Till I Collapse" by Eminem ft. Nate Dogg
This song is all about perseverance and pushing through, making it ideal for challenging workouts.

9. "Happy" by Pharrell Williams
A feel-good song that lifts your spirits and keeps you motivated throughout your exercise routine.

10. "Firework" by Katy Perry
An empowering anthem that encourages you to embrace your inner strength, perfect for any workout.

11. "Run the World (Girls)" by Beyoncé
A powerful track that boosts confidence and motivation, great for high-energy workouts.

12. "Pump It" by The Black Eyed Peas
With its fast-paced beat, this track is perfect for cardio and high-intensity workouts.

13. "Don't Stop Believin'" by Journey
A classic rock anthem that inspires perseverance and is perfect for the final stretch of your workout.

14. "We Will Rock You" by Queen
An iconic song with a powerful beat, great for strength training or any empowering workout..

15. "Gonna Be Alright" by Aneessa
Aneessa's uplifting and positive track is perfect for boosting your mood and motivation during your workout. Its feel-good vibe and catchy melody make it a great addition to any playlist.

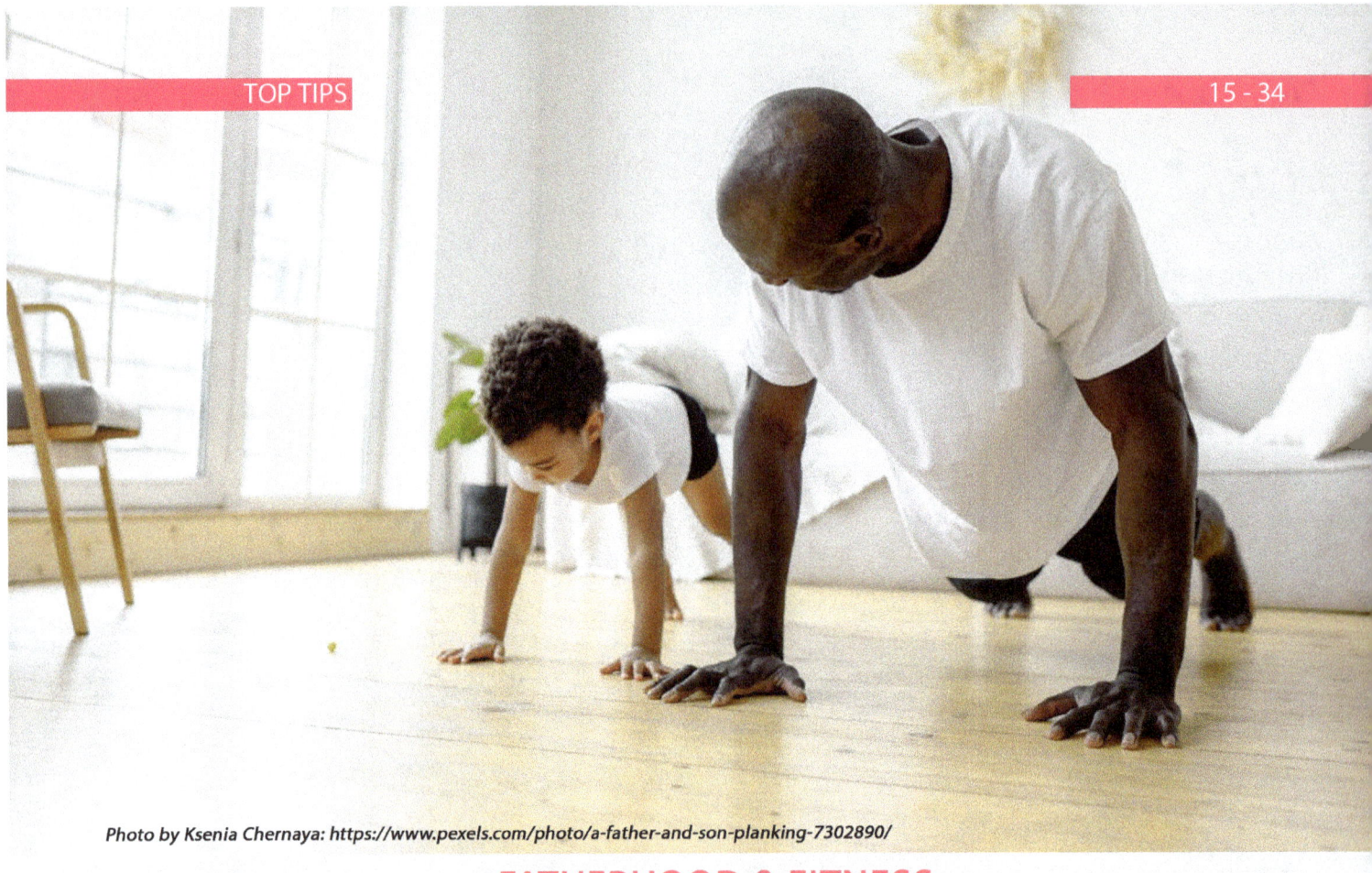

Photo by Ksenia Chernaya: https://www.pexels.com/photo/a-father-and-son-planking-7302890/

FATHERHOOD & FITNESS: BECOMING A STRONGER MAN FOR THE ONES WHO MATTER MOST

Being a father is one of the most rewarding and demanding roles a man can have. It's a daily commitment of love, protection, and leadership. But in the middle of sleepless nights, school drop-offs, work stress, and life's endless to-do list, one crucial thing often gets pushed aside—your health and fitness.

WHY FITNESS MATTERS FOR DADS

Fatherhood isn't just about being present—it's about being capable. When you're strong, energized, and mentally sharp, you're better equipped to chase your kids around the yard, carry them on your shoulders, and be the role model they need. Fitness improves your mood, builds resilience, and helps you stay disciplined—not just for the gym, but for life.

MENTAL HEALTH & WELLNESS: YOUR FAMILY NEEDS THE BEST VERSION OF YOU

Let's face it—fatherhood can be overwhelming. It's easy to bottle things up and carry the weight in silence. But your mental health is just as important as your physical strength.
Regular exercise helps combat stress, anxiety, and depression. More importantly, taking time for you—even just 20–30 minutes a day—can clear your head, improve your focus, and boost emotional resilience.

Don't be afraid to talk, open up, or ask for support. Real strength lies in knowing when to take care of your mind as much as your body. Meditation, journaling, therapy, or even quiet time in your garage gym can be powerful tools for self-care.

TRAIN FOR LIFE

Focus on functional strength—lifting, carrying, pushing, pulling—the kind of movement that mimics dad life. Add in cardio for heart health and mobility work to keep you pain-free as the kids grow. It's not about six-packs; it's about being present and powerful for your family.

For more inspiration, mental health resources, and fitness tips for busy dads,
Visit www.pumpitupmagazine.com
Want to share your journey? Email us at info@pumpitupmagazine.com

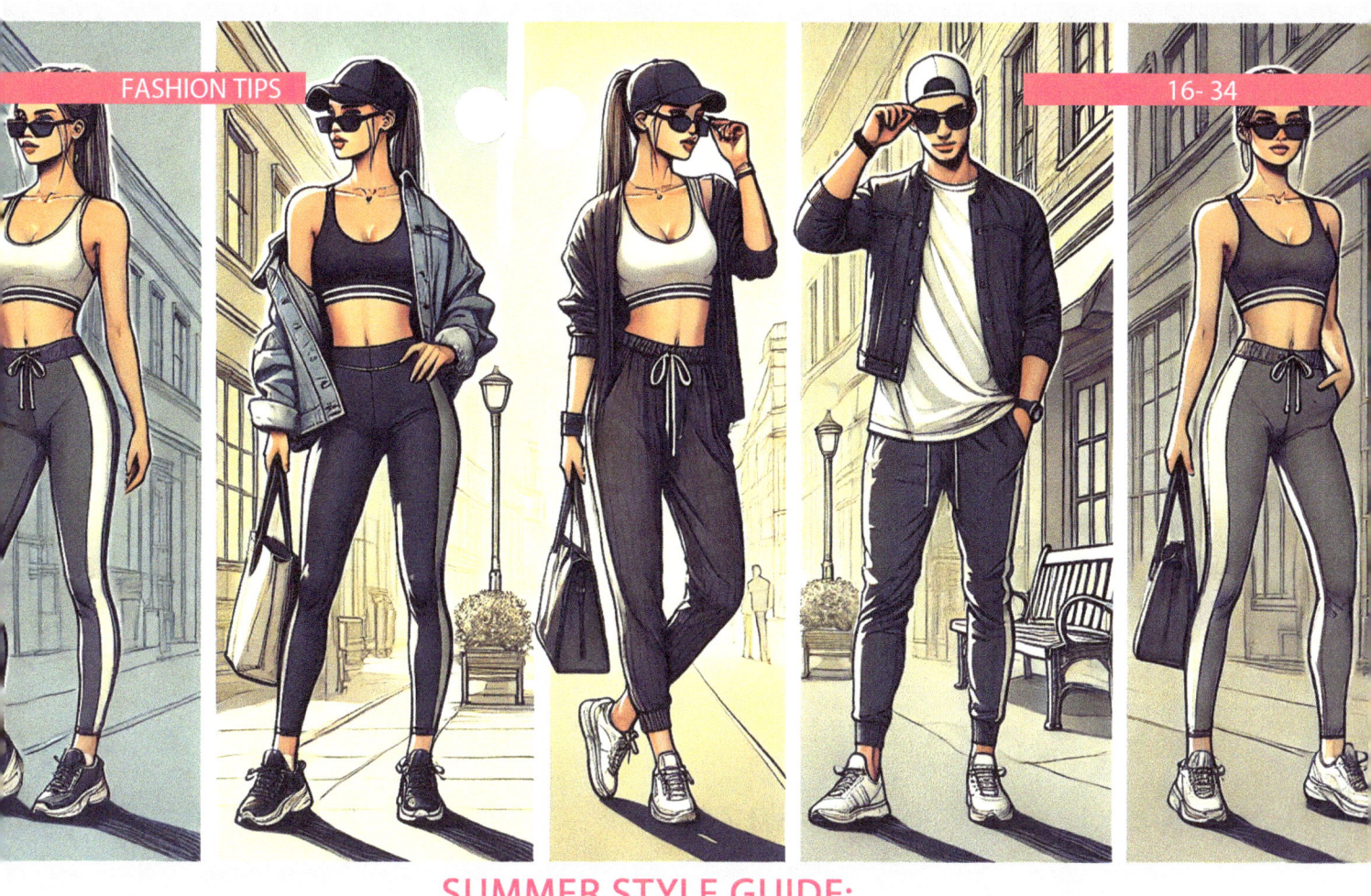

SUMMER STYLE GUIDE: FROM GYM TO STREET CHIC

Transitioning from a workout to a stylish street look is easy with the right pieces. This summer, the gym-to-street chic trend is both practical and fashionable. Here's how you can achieve it:

FOR WOMEN:

Start with Activewear: High-waisted leggings and a sports bra create a comfortable and flattering base.
Layer Up: Add a lightweight or denim jacket for an extra touch of style.
Accessories: Complete the look with a trendy cap, sunglasses, and a simple tote bag.
Footwear: Swap gym sneakers for trendy slip-on shoes to elevate your outfit.

FOR MEN:

Active Basics: Begin with athletic joggers and a fitted t-shirt.
Add Layers: A lightweight jacket like a bomber or hoodie can make the outfit street-ready.
Accessories: A cap and a sleek backpack add both style and functionality.
Footwear: Choose stylish sneakers for a polished look.

KEY POINTS:

Versatility: Choose pieces that work for both gym and casual settings.
Comfort & Style: Prioritize comfort while adding stylish touches.
Accessories Matter: Simple accessories can significantly enhance your look.

Embracing the gym-to-street chic trend means blending practicality with fashion.

With these tips, you can stay comfortable and stylish throughout the day, whether you're heading from the gym to a casual outing or running errands.

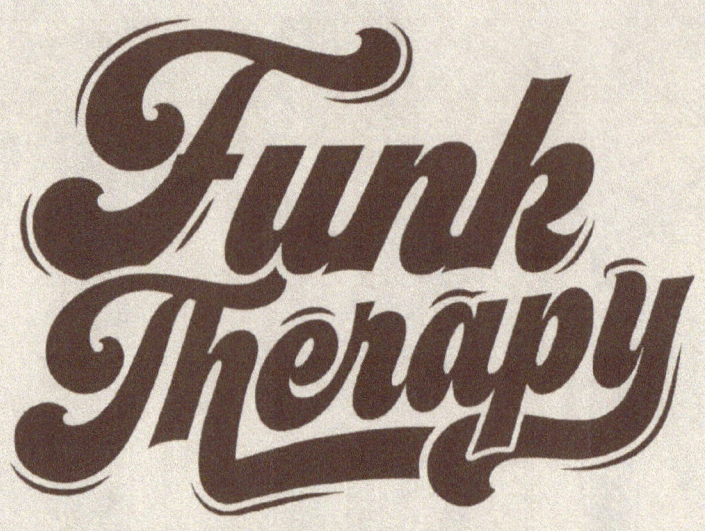

| Funky | Trendy | Cool | Hip |

Wear The Music You Love!

Visit our merchandise store on our website:

WWW.FUNKTHERAPYMUSIC.COM

10% Discount code: STAYFUNKY

- Hoodies
- Crop Top
- Sweat Pants
- Bucket Hats
- Slides
- Mugs

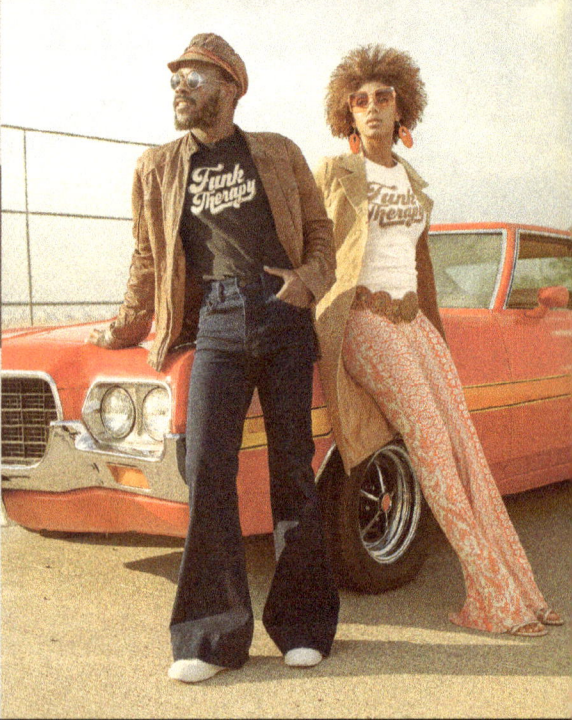

UNISEX T-SHIRTS

Brown T-Shirt
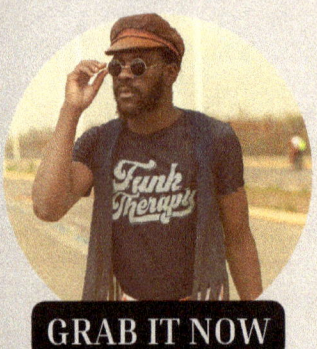
GRAB IT NOW

Orange T-Shirt
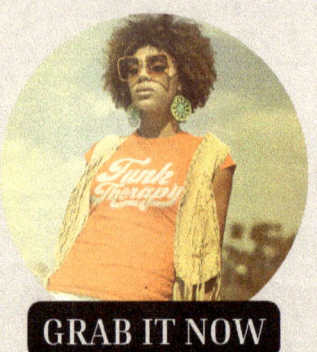
GRAB IT NOW

Beige T-Shirts
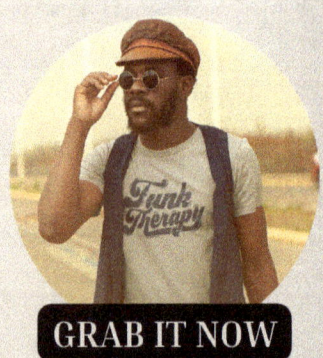
GRAB IT NOW

Join our community
@funktherapy2

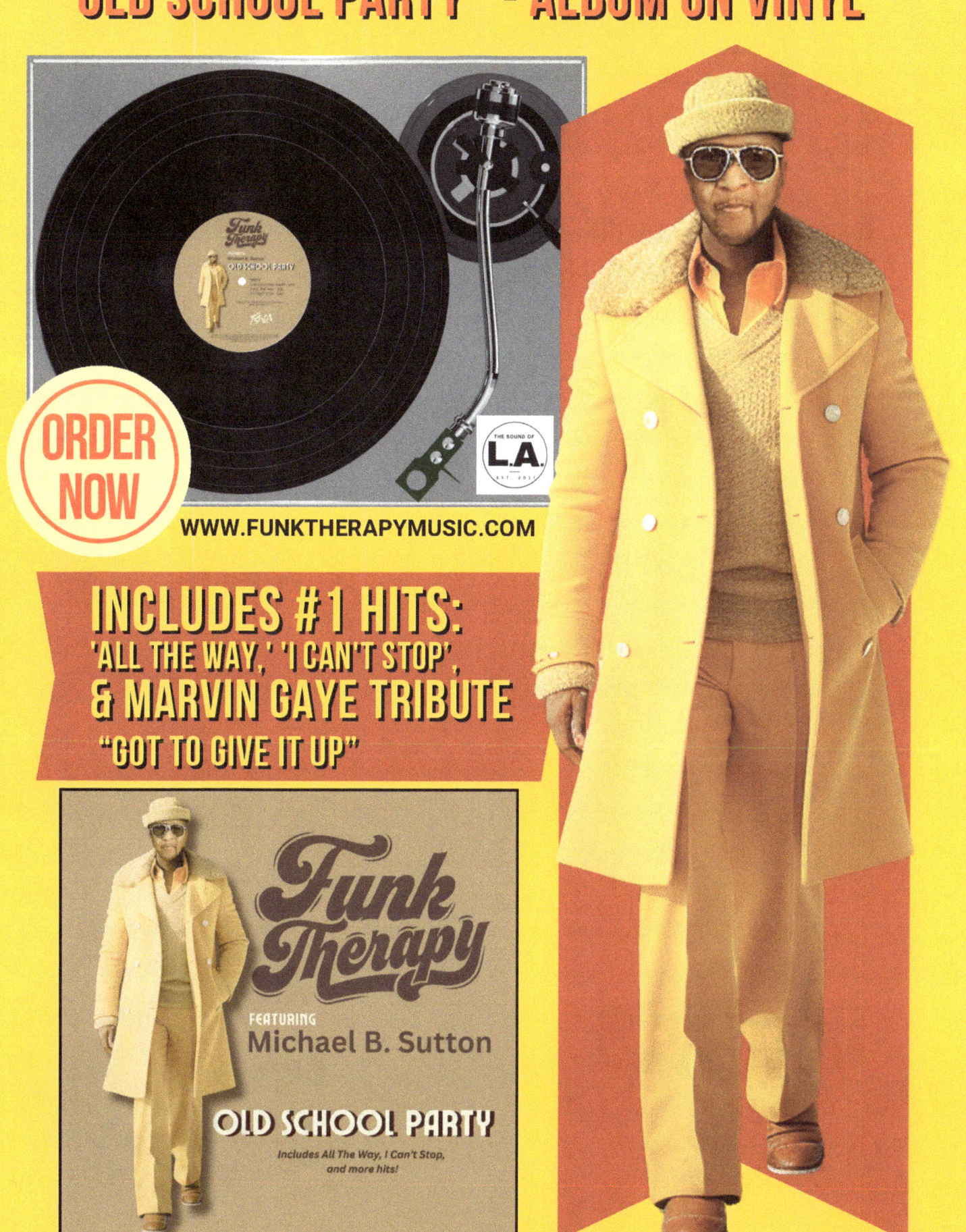

EXPLORE
The World

WHY YOU SHOULD CONSIDER TRAVELING IN A MOTOR HOME

Freedom

When you travel with a motor home, you have the ultimate freedom to explore the world. You can go wherever you want, when you want and stay as long as you desire. No need to worry about finding a place to stay, looking for public transportation or dealing with airline tickets!

Affordability

You'll save money on accommodation since you'll be staying in your own self-contained living space. You'll also save money on food costs since you'll have a fully functioning kitchen in your motor home. Not to mention, you'll save money on transport as your motor home will get you from point A to point B.

Comfort

You will have access to a full kitchen, living area, sleeping quarters and bathroom, all in one vehicle. This means that you won't have to worry about packing up your things each time you move from one place to another. Plus, you don't have to worry about expensive hotel bills when you stay on the road for long periods of time.

BOOK NOW

- 123981 Craftsman Rd., Calabasas, CA 91302
- 1(818) 225-8239
- www.expeditionmotorhomes.com/

WELLNESS TIPS

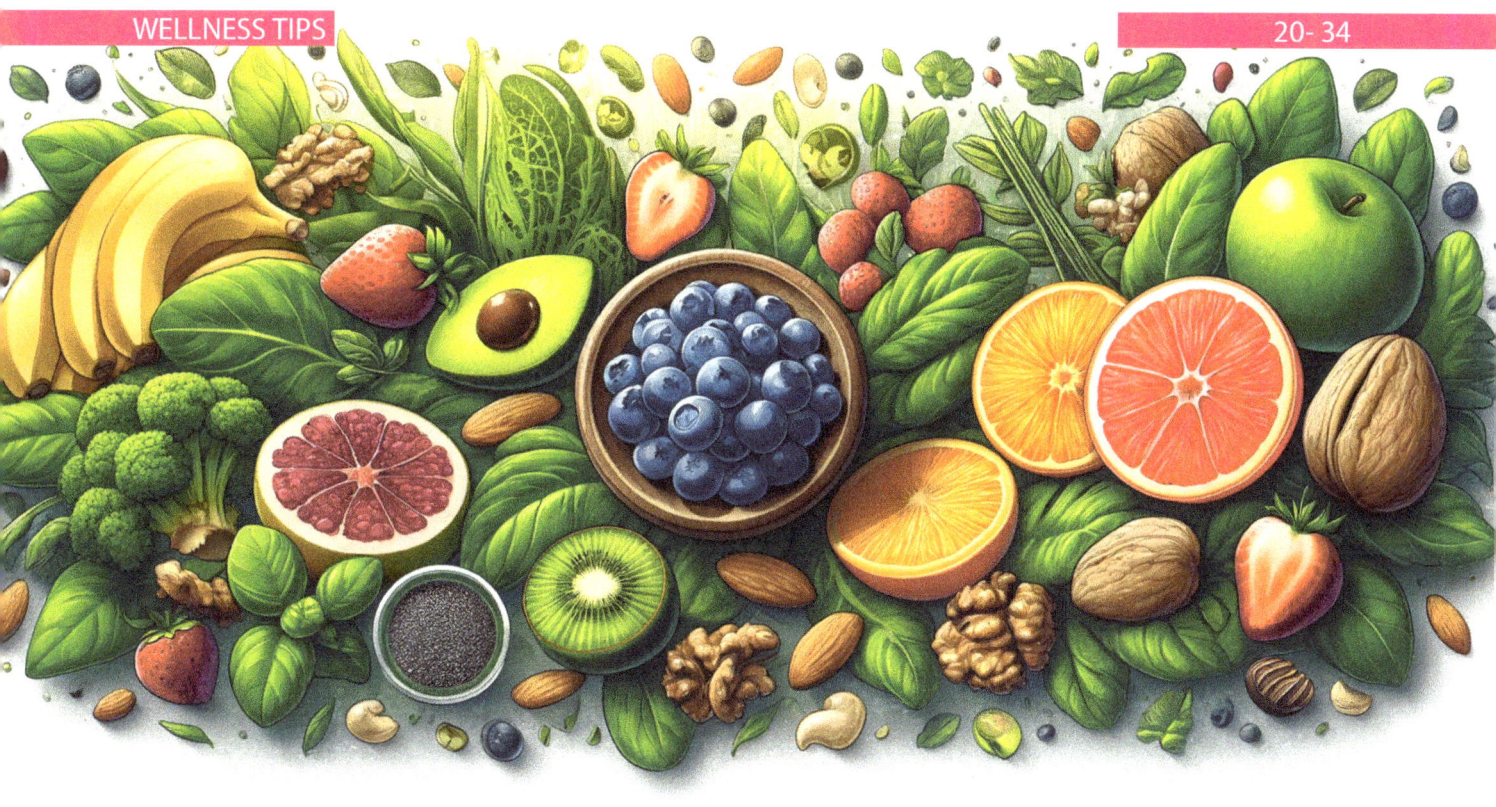

BEST SUPERFOODS FOR ENERGY & IMMUNITY

Boosting your energy levels and supporting your immune system can be achieved by incorporating superfoods into your diet. These nutrient-dense foods provide essential vitamins, minerals, and antioxidants that promote overall health. Here are some of the best superfoods to include in your diet:

1. BERRIES
Blueberries, strawberries, and raspberries are packed with antioxidants and vitamins, helping to protect against illness and boost energy levels.

2. SPINACH
Rich in iron and vitamin C, spinach enhances energy and supports a healthy immune system.

3. NUTS AND SEEDS
Almonds, walnuts, chia seeds, and flaxseeds are excellent sources of healthy fats, protein, and fiber. They provide sustained energy and essential nutrients.

4. CITRUS FRUITS
Oranges, lemons, and grapefruits are high in vitamin C, which is vital for immune function and skin health.

5. GREEN TEA
Loaded with antioxidants, green tea can boost metabolism and enhance immune function.

KEY BENEFITS:
Energy Boost: Superfoods provide sustained energy throughout the day.
Immune Support: Nutrient-rich foods strengthen the immune system.

Including these superfoods in your daily diet can help you stay energized and support your immune system, ensuring you feel your best every day.

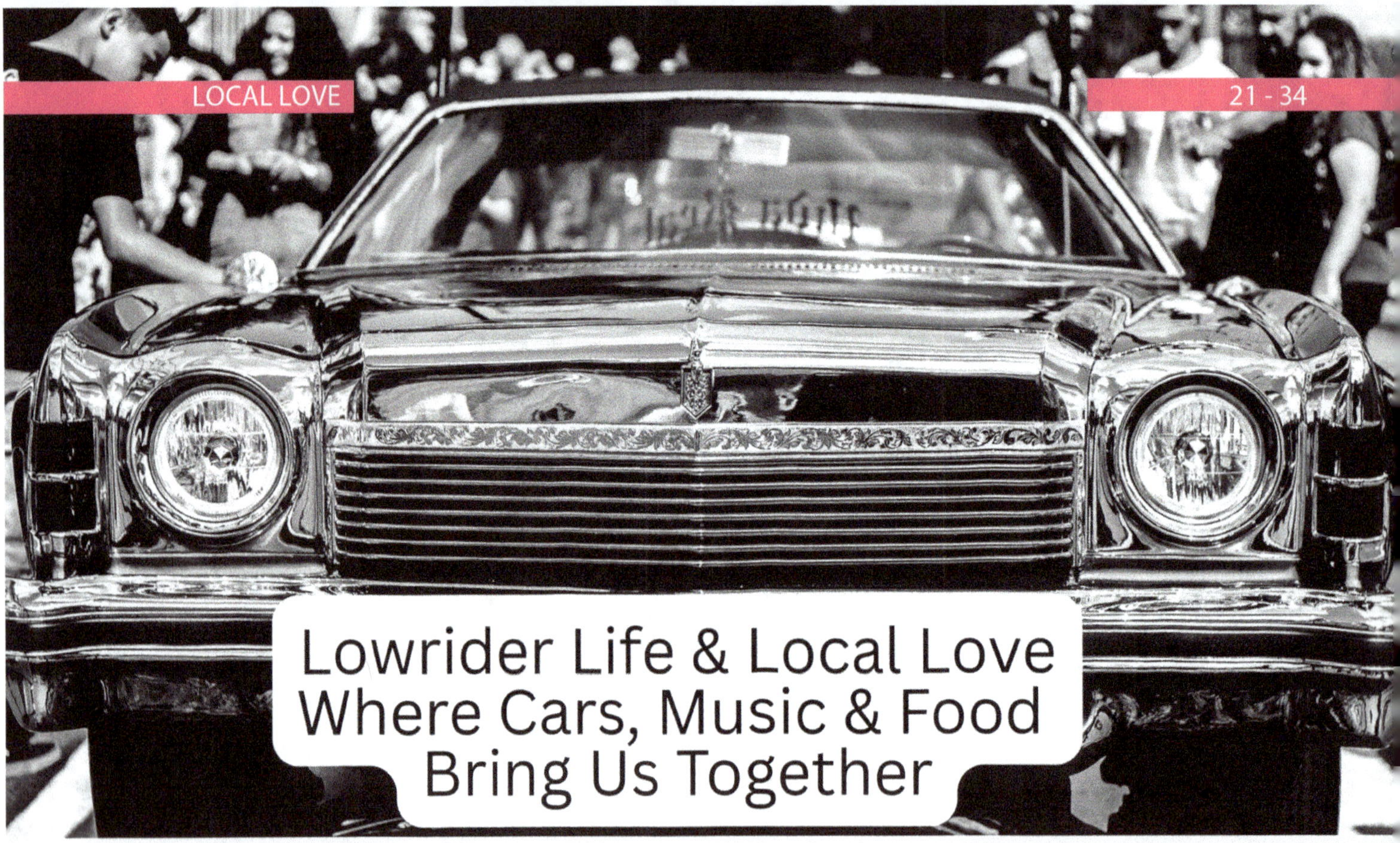

Lowrider Life & Local Love
Where Cars, Music & Food Bring Us Together

In the heart of our neighborhoods, something beautiful happens when chrome shines in the sun, oldies play on the speakers, and the smell of street tacos fills the air. This is more than a car scene—it's culture, community, and connection. Welcome to Lowrider Life.

THE ART OF THE LOWRIDER
A lowrider isn't just a car—it's a moving canvas. Every paint stroke, every hydraulic bounce, every chrome trim tells a story of pride, creativity, and heritage. Whether it's a candy-painted Impala or a meticulously restored Monte Carlo, lowriders represent art passed down through generations, blending style, soul, and self-expression.

LOCAL LOVE IN EVERY BLOCK
Lowrider gatherings aren't just car shows—they're family reunions. You'll see grandparents, kids, and teens all vibing together. These events unite local businesses, artists, and food vendors. From local DJs spinning classics to BBQ grills and food trucks dishing out comfort food, every detail reflects neighborhood pride.

MUSIC, MEMORIES & MOVEMENT
The soundtrack to Lowrider Life is smooth and timeless: Chicano soul, West Coast funk, old-school R&B. It's more than nostalgia—it's a reminder of who we are and where we come from. It brings healing, joy, and that undeniable bounce that moves your heart before your feet.

MORE THAN A TREND—IT'S A LIFESTYLE
Lowrider culture is rooted in resilience, love, and identity. It's about honoring our roots while celebrating the present—with a little flash, a lot of flavor, and whole lot of community love.

CRUISE TO THE SMOOTHEST LOWRIDER VIBES!
STREAM NOW: LOWRIDER LOVE PLAYLIST ON SPOTIFY
https://open.spotify.com/playlist/4MjPTPMVfgdF48S5phVTix

Cruise with us at www.pumpitupmagazine.com
Want to showcase your ride, business, or story?
Email info@pumpitupmagazine.com

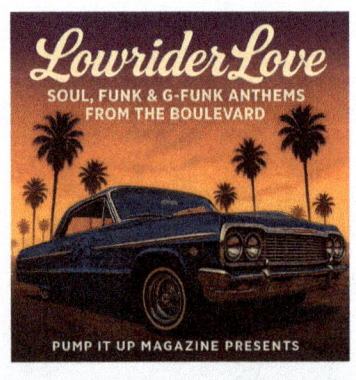

IRIE LOVE
Feel The Soul of the Queen of Island Reggae!
Sugah
Pump it up
"SUGAH"
WORLDSOUND AMERICAN ARTISTE
Virgin MUSIC GROUP
UNIVERSAL
NEW SINGLE AVAILABLE NOW
WWW.THISISIRIELOVE.COM

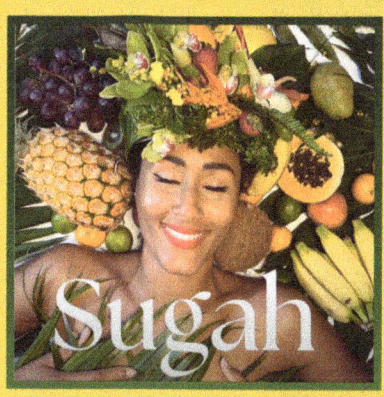

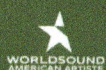

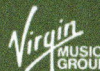

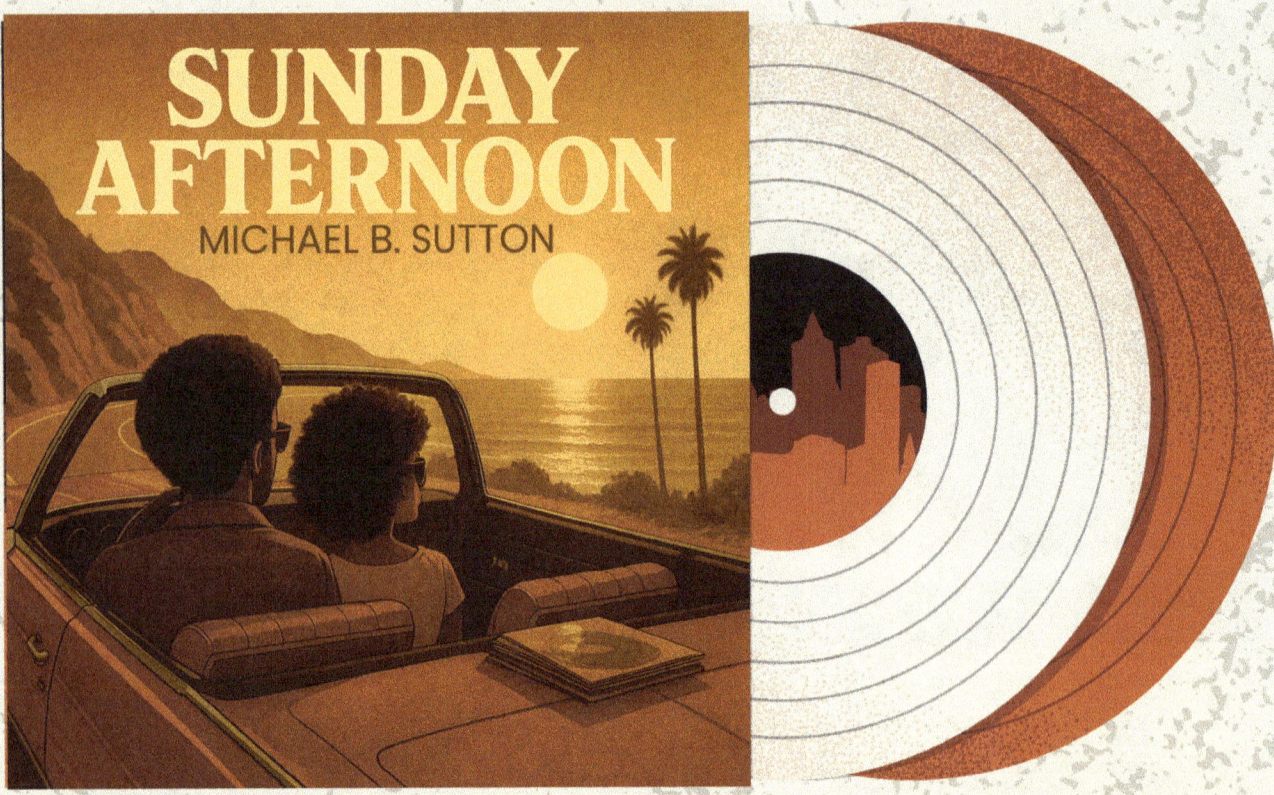

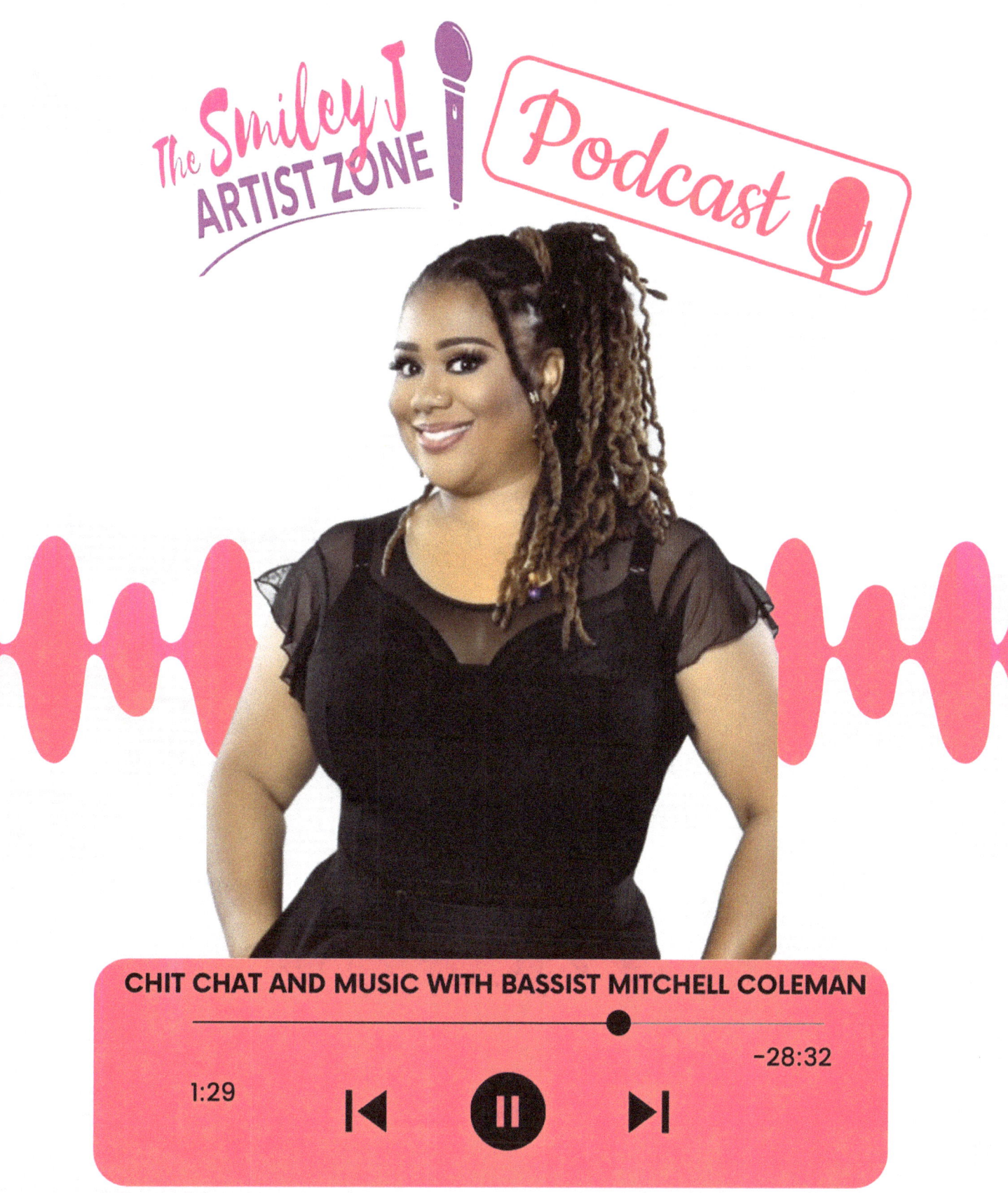

Listen to The Smiley J. Artist Zone
www.thesmileyjartistzone.podbean.com
and on all your favorite
streaming platforms!

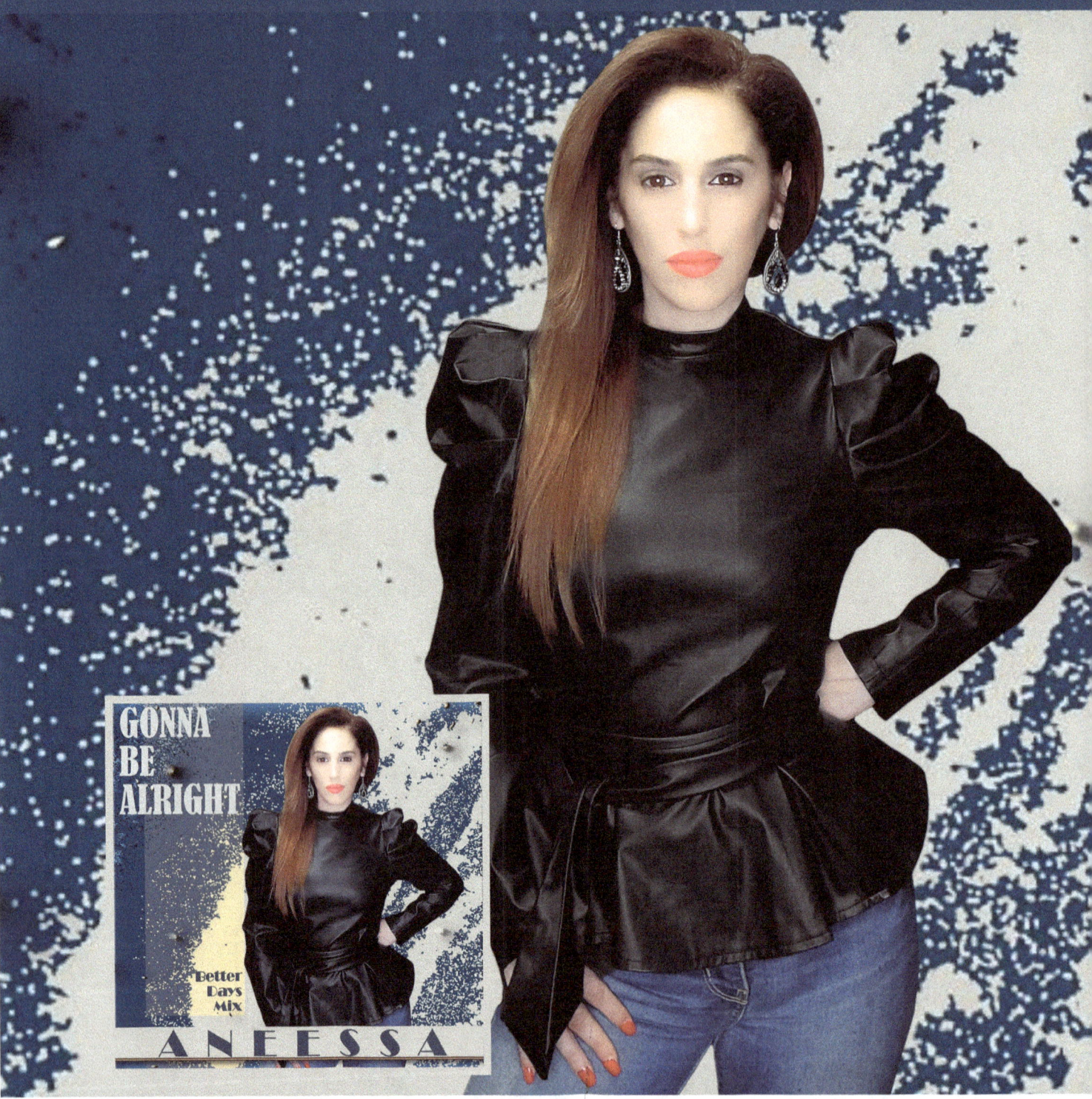

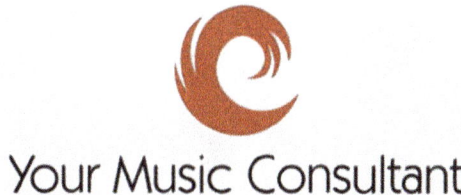

Your Music Consultant

Pump up Your Business!

1. Starter Launch Plan
For anyone with a dream but no legal setup yet
- ✅ 1-on-1 Discovery Call to map your path
- ✅ Help choosing the right structure (LLC, S-Corp, Sole Proprietor)
- ✅ EIN Registration (so you can get paid)
- ✅ Business Bank & Credit Guidance
- ✅ ASCAP/BMI Registration (for artists)
- ✅ Launch Checklist (PDF + Editable)

$897

💡 We explain everything in plain English — no business jargon needed.

2. Brand & Biz Builder
For those ready to go public & build credibility online
- ✅ Everything in Starter Launch
- ✅ 3 Social Media Pages Setup (IG, FB, LinkedIn or YouTube)
- ✅ Google Business Profile or YouTube Channel Setup
- ✅ Credit & DUNS Number Support
- ✅ Publishing or SEO Setup (depending on artist or business)
- ✅ 30-Day Social Launch Calendar
- ✅ Basic Website Starter (one-page scroll)

$2,500

3. Pro Website + Brand Launch
You want the full system — optimized, branded, and automated

- ✅ Everything in Builder
- ✅ Fully Custom, SEO-Optimized Website (3–5 pages)
- ✅ Custom Branding (Logo, Tagline, Brand Colors)
- ✅ Email Marketing Setup
- ✅ Royalty Mapping & Publishing Strategy (for artists)
- ✅ Personalized Growth Plan & Success Coaching

$3,500

⚠️ **PLEASE NOTE:**
Content creation, banner/post graphics, design materials, and social media posting are not included in these packages. 🎵 Custom videos, graphics, banners, and posting strategies are available for an additional fee.

→ **Book your free call today - Call now: +1 424-280-3119**
Visit ou website: www.yourmusicconsultant.com

Editions L.A.

DIGITAL CREATIVE AGENCY

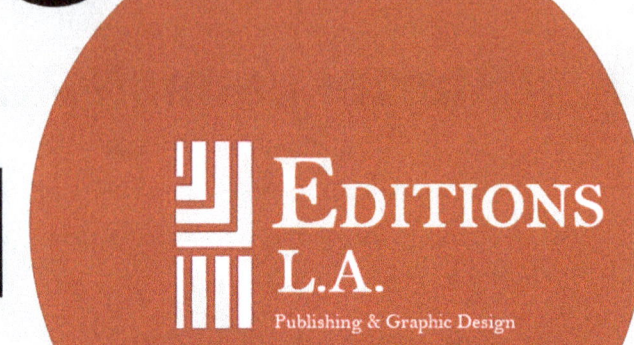

We Transform Your Vision Into Creative Results

Editions L.A. is a full-service agency based in Los Angeles. Our company is a collective of amazing people striving to build delightful services
We believe that is all about getting your message across clearly and with a "Wow!" thrown in for good measure.

Our Awesome Services

Branding

We build, style and tone your brand identity from the ground up.
We rebrand established bands, brands or businesses.

Merchandise Store
Website design and E-Commerce
Website updates

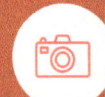

Digital Marketing

CD Cover | Banners | Logo design | Flyers | Brochures | Leaflets | Print ads | Magazine covers & artworks
Facebook / twitter / instagram / youtube artworks | Book cover
Infographics | Icon Design |
| TshirtsProduct Labels | Presentation slides
Corporate graphics
Professional photo editing & enhancing
Redesign existing elements
YouTube Optimization and Monetization
Youtube Video Editing
Lyric Video and Advertising Design.

Publishing

BOOK COVER DESIGN
EBOOK FORMATTING SERVICES
and distribution on major platforms
(Amazon, Barnes & Nobles..)

Tell us about your dream and we will make it true!

Editions L.A.
7210 Jordan Avenue Suite B42, Canoga Park, California 91303, United States
info@edtions-la.com
Website: www.editions-la.com

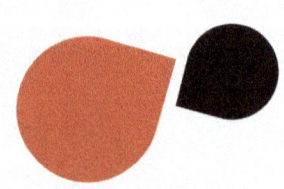

HOW TO DEAL WITH TOXIC PEOPLE

1. RECOGNIZE WHAT MAKES YOU AN EASY PREY

Is it often your fear of rocking the boat or the need to please them that keeps you tongue-tied when your "friend" takes it out on you. Use rational thinking to process the interactions you have had with the friend that made you unhappy. Focus on why you felt what you did, not what you felt, and try to decipher if you can get a pattern.

2. MOVE ON WITHOUT THEM

If you know a friend who always destructively dictates the emotional atmosphere, be sure of this – they are toxic. If you are suffering because of a person's attitude, and your patience, advice, compassion, and attentiveness do not seem to help them, and they don't seem to care a bit, ask yourself, "Do I really need this human in my life?" When you remove toxic people from your life, it becomes way easier to breathe.

3. PUT YOUR FOOT DOWN

Your dignity may be ravaged, attacked, and mocked, but it can never be taken away from you unless you surrender it willingly. It is all about finding the self-love to defend your boundaries. Make it clear that you won't allow anyone to insult or belittle you. You can effectively end conversations that are putting you down with plain abruptness or sickening sweetness. The message should be clear – you will entertain no games.

4. STOP ACCEPTING THEIR TOXIC BEHAVIOR

Toxic people often use their moody and loud behavior to get preferential treatment. You may find it easier to quiet them down by giving in to their demands than listen to their nagging. Don't be fooled into doing this.

Short-term comfort will equal long-term headache for you in a situation like this. Toxic people won't change if they get rewarded for not changing. Constant negativity and drama are never worth putting up with.

5. SPEAK UP

Stand up for yourself. Some people can do anything for their personal gain at the expense of others – take your money and property, pass guilt, cut in line, bully and belittle others, etc. Do not accept this kind of behavior. These people know what they are doing is wrong. They will back down considerably quickly when confronted. In most social settings, people tend to be quiet until one person speaks up. So, speak up!

6. PRACTICE PRACTICAL COMPASSION

You aren't really helping someone by accepting everything they do just because they have issues. There are a lot of people who go through extreme hardships, but they are not toxic to others around them. We can only be genuinely compassionate when we set respectful boundaries. Making too many allowances and pardons is not healthy for anyone in the long-term. Always remember, even people with clinical/mental illnesses or legitimate problems can comprehend that you may have your own needs as well, which means you need to politely excuse yourself when you feel things are getting out of hand. You deserve this 'me' time. You deserve to live peacefully, free from toxic behavior and external pressure, with no boundaries to uphold, problems to solve, or people to please.

QUIZ

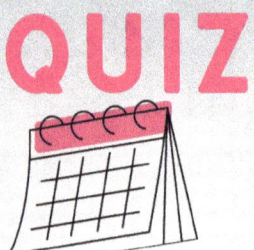

Test Your Mental Strength

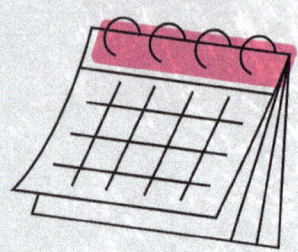

1. What do you do to manage stress?
- A) EXERCISE
- B) MEDITATE
- C) TALK TO A FRIEND
- D) ALL OF THE ABOVE

2. How often do you take time for yourself?
- A) DAILY
- B) WEEKLY
- C) MONTHLY
- D) RARELY

3. What's your go-to activity when you need a mental break?
- A) READING A BOOK
- B) TAKING A WALK
- C) WATCHING A MOVIE
- D) OTHER: _____

4. How do you practice mindfulness?
- A) MEDITATION
- B) DEEP BREATHING EXERCISES
- C) JOURNALING
- D) I DON'T PRACTICE MINDFULNESS

5. How do you feel about seeking help from a mental health professional?
- A) VERY COMFORTABLE
- B) SOMEWHAT COMFORTABLE
- C) UNCOMFORTABLE
- D) HAVEN'T THOUGHT ABOUT IT

6. What's one thing you do to stay positive?
- A) POSITIVE AFFIRMATIONS
- B) GRATITUDE JOURNALING
- C) SURROUNDING MYSELF WITH POSITIVE PEOPLE
- D) OTHER: _____

7. How often do you check in with your emotions?
- A) DAILY
- B) WEEKLY
- C) MONTHLY
- D) RARELY

8. How do you cope with feeling overwhelmed?
- A) TAKE A BREAK
- B) TALK TO SOMEONE
- C) ENGAGE IN A HOBBY
- D) OTHER: _____

Scoring:

Mostly A's: Mental Strength Champion
You have excellent mental strength and prioritize your mental health. Keep up the great work and continue practicing these healthy habits!

Mostly B's: Mentally Strong with Room to Grow
You have good mental strength but could benefit from incorporating more self-care practices. Try adding a few new strategies to your routine.

Mostly C's: Building Your Mental Strength
You're on the right track but might need more consistent mental health practices. Focus on making self-care a regular part of your life.

Mostly D's: Needs Improvement
It looks like you might struggle with maintaining mental strength. Consider seeking support from a mental health professional and trying new self-care techniques.

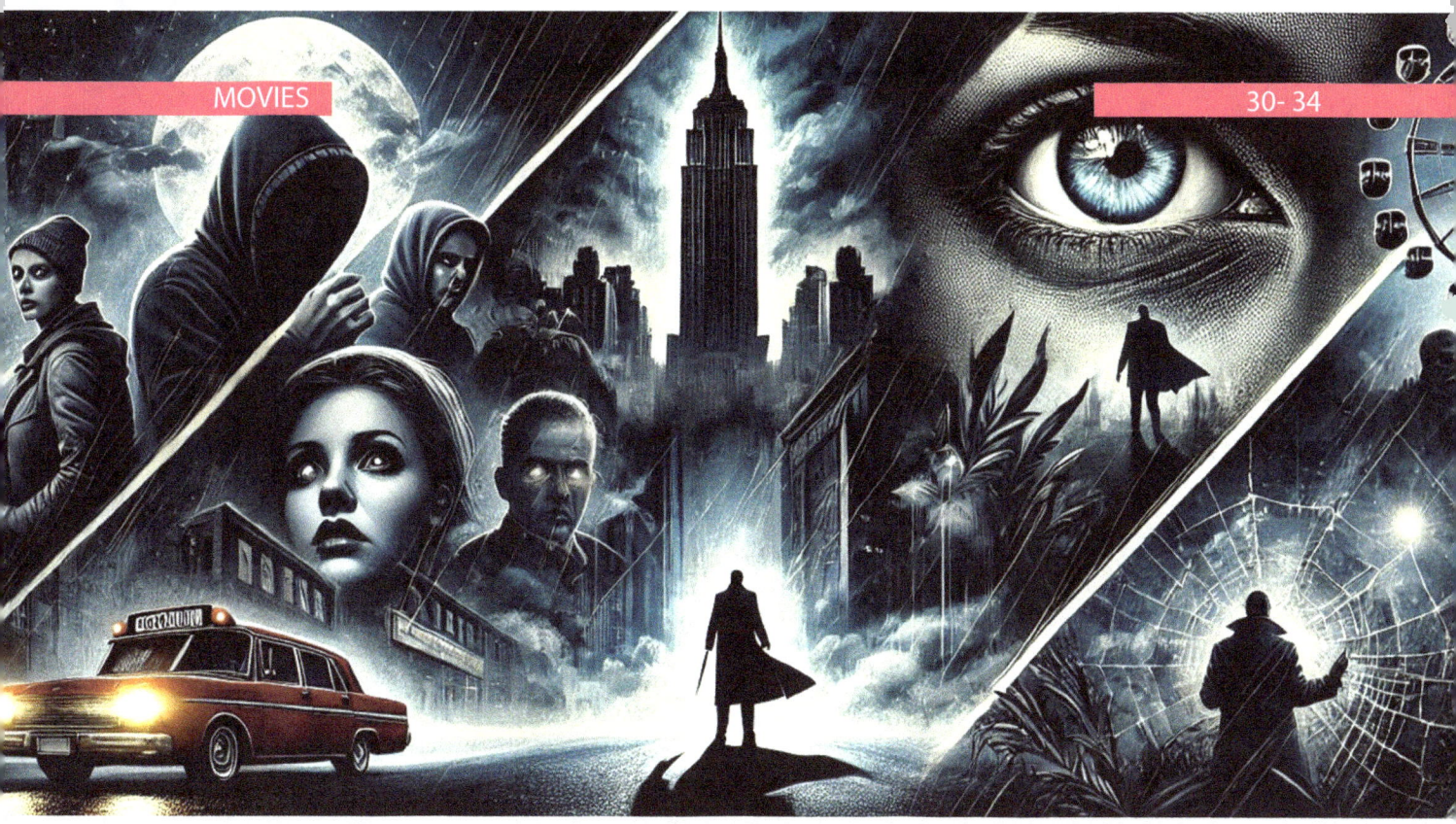

BEST THRILLERS
TO KEEP YOU ON THE EDGE OF YOUR SEAT

1. "FIGHT CLUB" (1999)
Directed by David Fincher and based on the novel by Chuck Palahniuk, "Fight Club" stars Edward Norton as an insomniac office worker who forms an underground fight club with the charismatic Tyler Durden, played by Brad Pitt. The film explores themes of identity, consumerism, and rebellion, culminating in a shocking twist that has become iconic.

2. "SE7EN" (1995)
Another masterpiece by David Fincher, "Se7en" follows detectives (Brad Pitt and Morgan Freeman) on the hunt for a serial killer who uses the seven deadly sins as motifs for his crimes. The film's dark, atmospheric setting and unexpected ending make it a gripping thriller.

3. "THE SILENCE OF THE LAMBS" (1991)
This classic thriller features Jodie Foster as FBI trainee Clarice Starling, who seeks the help of Dr. Hannibal Lecter (Anthony Hopkins), an imprisoned cannibalistic serial killer, to catch another killer. The film is renowned for its intense psychological interplay and unforgettable performances.

4. "GONE GIRL" (2014)
Directed by David Fincher and based on the novel by Gillian Flynn, "Gone Girl" tells the story of a man who becomes the prime suspect in his wife's disappearance. The movie is known for its twists and turns, exploring themes of media manipulation and marital deception.

5. "INCEPTION" (2010)
Christopher Nolan's "Inception" is a mind-bending thriller that delves into the realm of dreams. Leonardo DiCaprio stars as a thief who enters people's dreams to steal secrets. The film's complex narrative structure and visually stunning scenes make it an exhilarating watch.

These films offer a mix of psychological depth, suspense, and unexpected twists, making them must-watch thrillers for anyone looking to experience gripping and thought-provoking cinema.

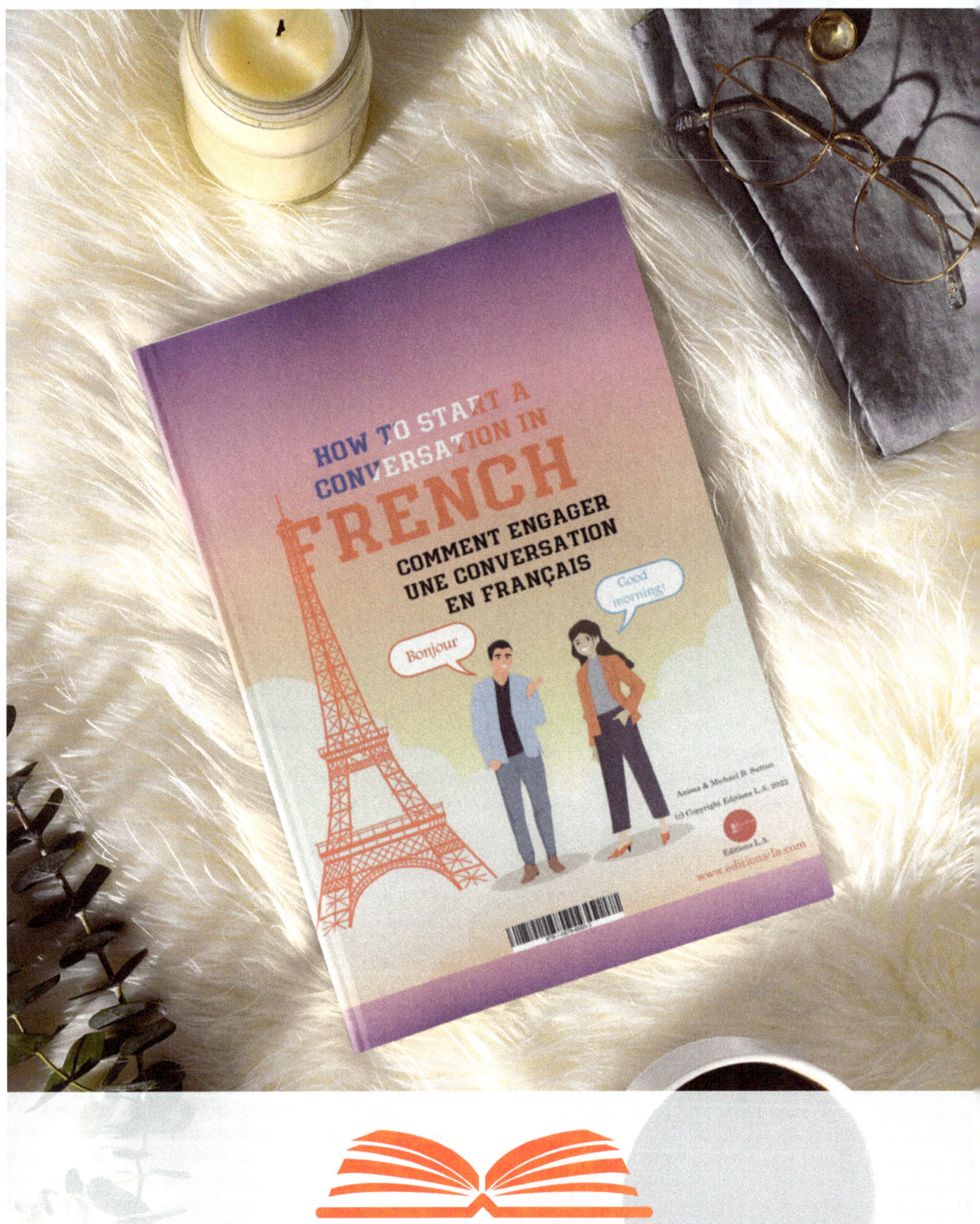

AWARENESS

DRIVE & DONATE:
EASY WAYS TO SHOW LOVE & SUPPORT
SUPPORT ARTISTS, UPLIFT COMMUNITIES, AND MAKE A DIFFERENCE.

Whether you're into custom cars, music, or local street art, there's a powerful way you can give back. Here are simple ways to support artists like Solo Element and other creatives who inspire us:

1. SHARE THEIR STORY
You don't have to spend money to show support. One of the easiest and most powerful things you can do is share an artist's work on social media.
Whether it's a post about a custom car, a clip of their process, or an article (like this one!) — that one share could land them a customer, a new fan, or a feature.
Tag your friends, repost their videos, and leave a kind comment.
It costs $0 to support someone's dream.

2. SHOW UP
Custom car events, pop-up shows, mural unveilings, community art walks — artists often pour their energy into creating experiences, not just content.
Your presence matters.
Whether it's a local lowrider cruise night or a gallery feature, showing up shows them you care. Plus, it connects you to the heartbeat of the community.

3. SHOP SMALL, BUY ART
That hoodie with original art. That vinyl with a handmade cover. That airbrushed canvas or painted skateboard deck.
When you buy from an artist, you're not just purchasing a product — you're investing in a person.
Your purchase might fund their next piece, pay for supplies, or help them pay rent.

4. DONATE TO A LOCAL CAUSE
Many artists partner with local charities, mental health awareness events, or youth programs.
At custom car shows, it's not uncommon to see raffles and fundraisers benefiting local schools, shelters, or medical causes.
Next time you attend a show or art market, ask where the proceeds go — your ticket or tip might help save a life.

5. VOLUNTEER YOUR TIME OR SKILL
If you're a photographer, designer, video editor, writer, or have business skills — you might be sitting on a resource that could elevate an artist to the next level.
Offer to help with a logo, build a website, or shoot behind-the-scenes footage.
If you don't have creative skills, just volunteering to help at an event or connect them with someone in your network can make a difference.

6. CELEBRATE THEM OUT LOUD
Leave a review. Nominate them for awards. Tell your friends.
A kind word, a repost, a shout-out in your story… those little ripples create real waves.
Artists and creatives often work behind the scenes, quietly battling doubt, burnout, or financial stress.
Your encouragement might be the boost they didn't know they needed that day.

♥ SUPPORT IS LOVE IN ACTION
Whether you're cheering from your phone or showing up front row — supporting your community doesn't have to be complicated.
It starts with one decision: to care.
Let's keep the wheels turning and the love flowing.

FRENCH
ENGLISH

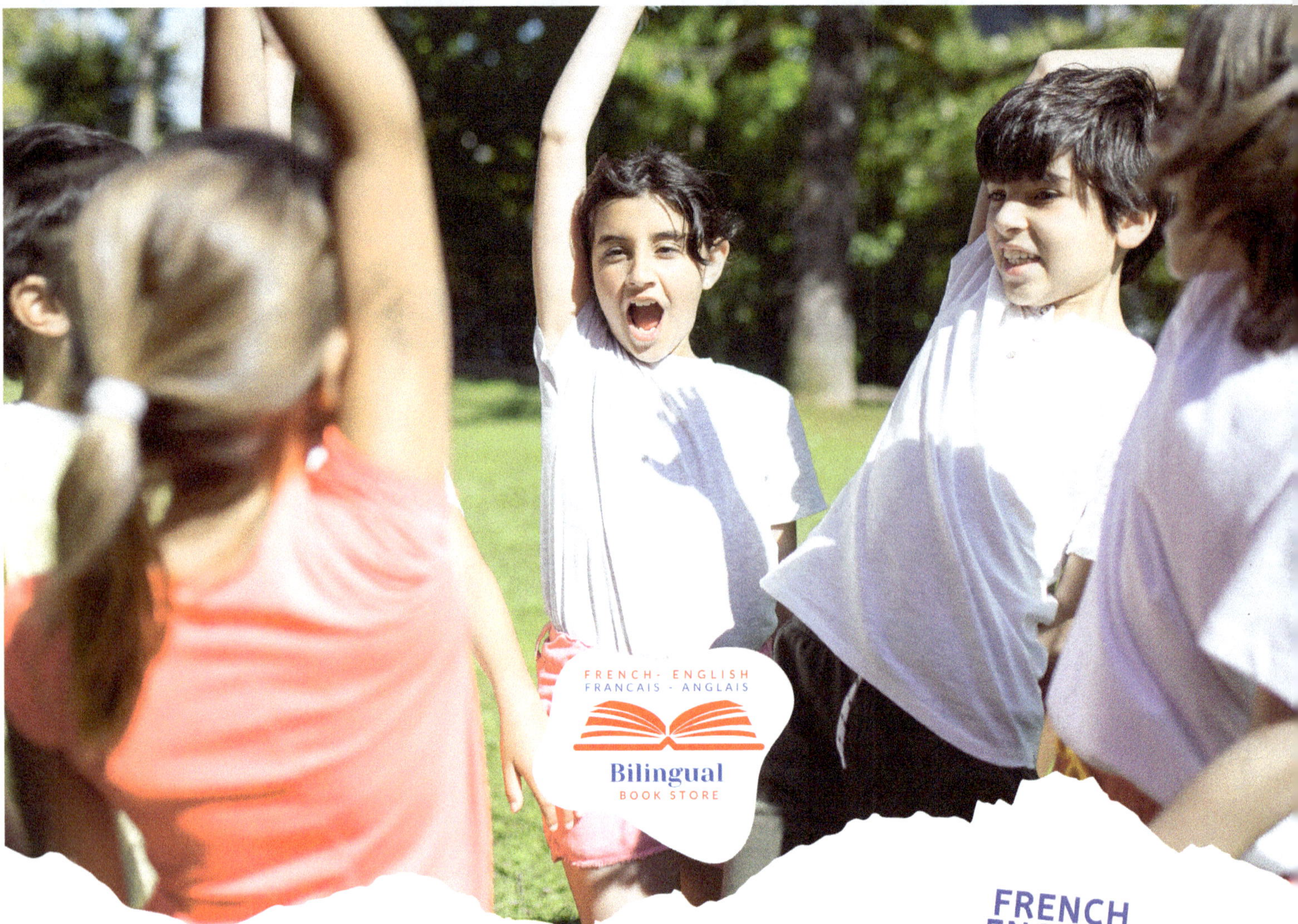

I AM - JE SUIS

AFFIRMATIONS POUR LA PENSÉE POSITIVE
AFFIRMATIONS FOR POSITIVE THINKING

Color & Learn French with Every Page!

Benefits

- Bilingual Skills: Get a head start on French and English.
- Positive Thinking: Helps kids see the bright side.
- Confidence Boost: Full of confidence-building affirmations.
- Fun Learning: Who knew coloring could teach you a language?
- Creativity Kick: Boosts those creative and motor skills.
- Smarter Every Day: Sharpens memory and helps kids multitask.
- Worldly Wise: Opens up a world of cultures.
- Family Time: Perfect for some fun learning together.
- Invest in the Future: Sets kids up for success down the road.

nook kobo INGRAM BARNES&NOBLE BOOKSELLERS iBooks amazon.com

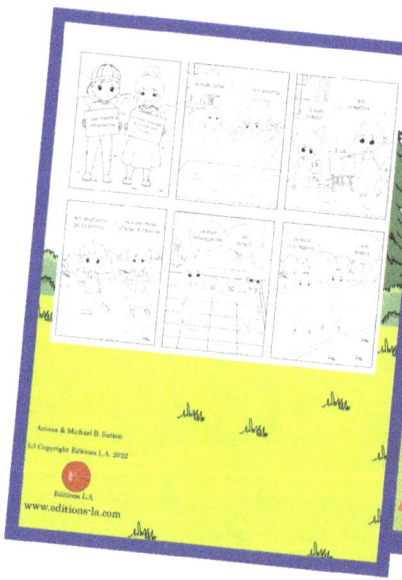

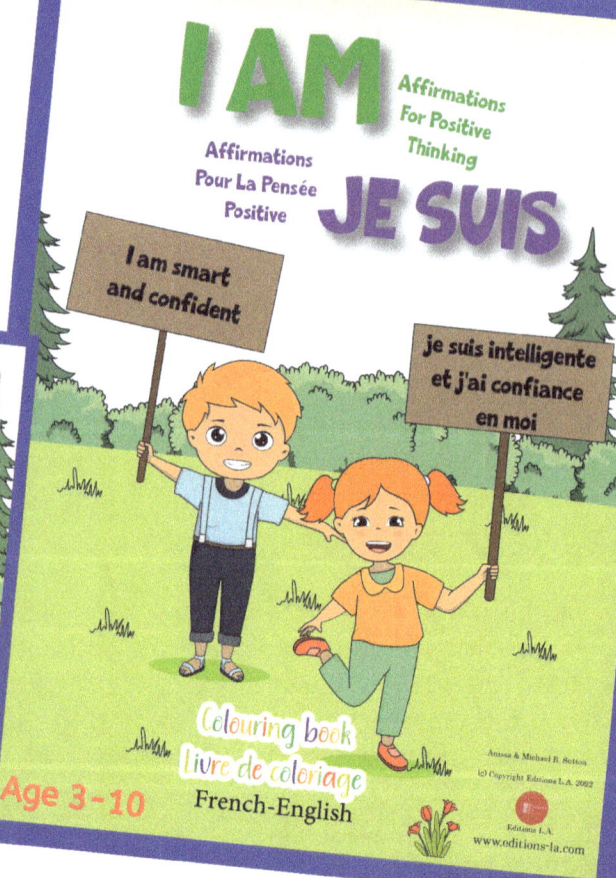

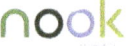

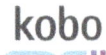

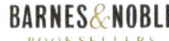

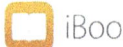

WWW.BILINGUALBOOKSTORE.COM

www.ingramcontent.com/pod-product-compliance
Lightning Source LLC
LaVergne TN
LVHW082245060526
838201LV00052B/1822